Second Wind

The Rise of the Ageless Athlete

Lee Bergquist

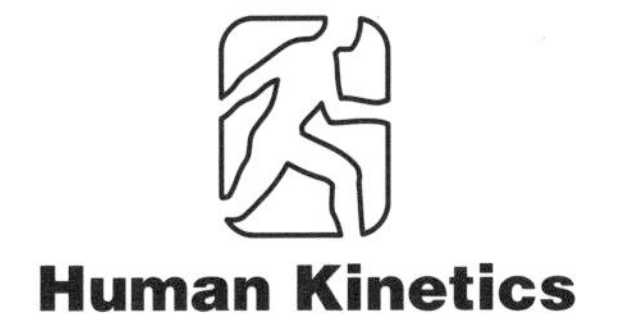

Human Kinetics

Second Wind

The Rise of the Ageless Athlete

Library of Congress Cataloging-in-Publication Data

Bergquist, Lee.
Second wind : the rise of the ageless athlete / Lee Bergquist.
p. cm.
Includes bibliographical references and index.
ISBN-13: 978-0-7360-7491-9 (soft cover)
ISBN-10: 0-7360-7491-0 (soft cover)
1. Sports for older people--Anecdotes. 2. Physical fitness for older people--Anecdotes. I. Title.
GV708.5.B47 2009
796.084'6--dc22
2009006759

ISBN-10: 0-7360-7491-0 (print)
ISBN-13: 978-0-7360-7491-9 (print)
ISBN-10: 0-7360-8523-8 (Adobe PDF)
ISBN-13: 978-0-7360-8523-6 (Adobe PDF)

The Web addresses cited in this text were current as of March 2009, unless otherwise noted.

Acquisitions Editor: Myles Schrag; **Developmental Editor:** Anne Hall; **Assistant Editor:** Cory Weber; **Copyeditor:** Jan Feeney; **Proofreader:** Anne Rogers; **Indexer:** Dan Connolly; **Permission Manager:** Martha Gullo; **Graphic Designer:** Joe Buck; **Graphic Artist:** Francine Hamerski and Tara Welsch; **Cover Designer:** Keith Blomberg; **Photographer (cover):** © Veronika Lukasova; **Photographer (interior):** Lee Bergquist, unless otherwise noted; **Photo Asset Manager:** Laura Fitch; **Visual Production Assistant:** Joyce Brumfield; **Photo Production Manager:** Jason Allen; **Printer:** McNaughton & Gunn

Human Kinetics books are available at special discounts for bulk purchase. Special editions or book excerpts can also be created to specification. For details, contact the Special Sales Manager at Human Kinetics.

Printed in the United States of America 10 9 8 7 6 5 4 3 2 1

The paper in this book is certified under a sustainable forestry program.

Human Kinetics
Web site: www.HumanKinetics.com

United States: Human Kinetics
P.O. Box 5076
Champaign, IL 61825-5076
800-747-4457
e-mail: humank@hkusa.com

Canada: Human Kinetics
475 Devonshire Road Unit 100
Windsor, ON N8Y 2L5
800-465-7301 (in Canada only)
e-mail: info@hkcanada.com

Europe: Human Kinetics
107 Bradford Road
Stanningley
Leeds LS28 6AT, United Kingdom
+44 (0) 113 255 5665
e-mail: hk@hkeurope.com

Australia: Human Kinetics
57A Price Avenue
Lower Mitcham, South Australia 5062
08 8372 0999
e-mail: info@hkaustralia.com

New Zealand: Human Kinetics
Division of Sports Distributors NZ Ltd.
P.O. Box 300 226 Albany
North Shore City
Auckland
0064 9 448 1207
e-mail: info@humankinetics.co.nz

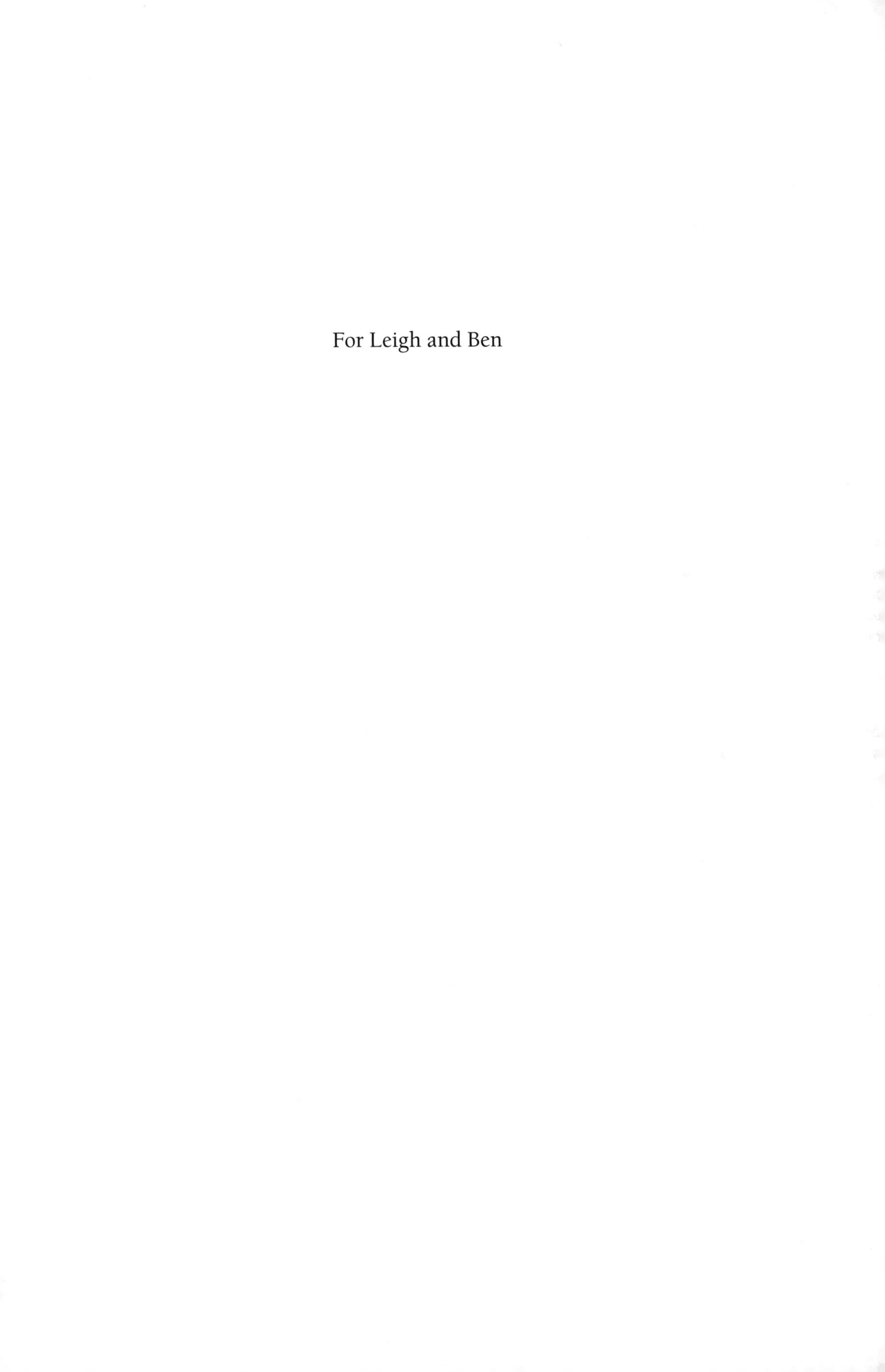

For Leigh and Ben

Contents

Acknowledgments

I owe a debt of gratitude to Rick Romell, whose careful reading vastly improved the manuscript; James B. Nelson, who offered guidance and encouragement from the beginning; and David Luce, who is five years older than me—and always in better shape.

I would also like to thank Peter Annin, Chuck Botsford, Gail Boxrud, Thomas Content, Ellen Gabler, G.D. Gearino, Jim Higgins, Annysa Johnson, Payton Jordan, Becky Lang, Greg Pearson, Phillip J. Ramthun, Mike Ruby, Ken Stone, and Bob Zahn for their help. Editor Marty Kaiser and managing editor George Stanley of the *Milwaukee Journal Sentinel* graciously provided me two leaves of absence for research and writing. This book would not be possible without the support of Rainer Martens, Myles Schrag, and Anne Hall at Human Kinetics. My agent, Neil Salkind, a competitive masters swimmer, immediately recognized the value of the project. Finally, I am forever grateful to my wife, Leigh Albritton, and son, Ben, for their love and encouragement.

Prologue

Sprinting Into Midlife

There was a time after I turned 40 when jogging became as tedious as a long car ride. My runs fell flat. My weekly mileage—never high in the first place—began to slip. I needed to move in a new direction, and since speed is associated with youth, I started running as fast as I could. In middle age, it's turned out to be one of the best decisions in my life.

Nine-year-olds can suddenly get up from the grass and run effortlessly across the yard. But adults who try to chase them usually move in slow motion. The body simply conspires to slow down as we age. We're told that lean muscle mass peaks at 25 and the heart and lungs reach their apex during our 30s. Then the slide begins. Muscles lose their flexibility. Bones become more brittle. Cells can't process oxygen as well. Eventually, the inner ear begins to erode so that little by little coordination suffers. These metabolic paper cuts can go unnoticed for years until one day we look in the mirror and ask ourselves, "Who the hell is that?"

Exercise will hold back our inevitable deterioration. In the coming years I would observe this repeatedly. I literally had to learn how to run fast again, since a flat-out sprint is a life skill that is normally forgotten by the time we're 18. I never ran track, so I had little basic knowledge to guide me. It took months of miscues and pulled muscles for my body to adapt and shift gears from endurance to speed. My watch was telling me I was getting faster. But how fast? You can jog forever and never stir a competitive fire. But when you run fast, you want to know how you'll match up. One year later I found myself on a starting line. My competitors had thinning hair and bulging quadriceps. They were all business. They looked like gunslingers ready to do each other in. Afterward, the tension evaporated. Everyone was smiling, shaking hands, and checking their times.

Sprinting introduced me to the intersecting worlds of aging and athleticism and a certain subculture known as masters athletics—the commonly accepted term for men and women who compete against people their own age. Masters competitions usually begin at the age of 40. Depending on the sport, the ranks build in numbers until age 60 when sickness, injuries, and lethargy start to weed people out. But not everyone. Some of the most fascinating people I've met are athletes in their 70s and 80s. They are the fortunate few with the health and fire in their bellies to keep going.

Some masters athletes are as driven as ambitious executives. But many simply find that an athletic act, executed with old bones and muscle, can give meaning to life in ways that love and religion cannot. They're a different breed, since even basic exercise has become a memory for too many Americans. Still, in many ways, older athletes are no different from their contemporaries. Some are filled with confidence. Others are riddled with doubt. Some use the games they play for friendship and camaraderie. Others find it a sanctuary from the rest of their lives. Most hope their conditioning will stretch out their active years—and maybe even let them live longer. They are cranky and fun loving, laconic and eloquent, generous and mistrusting, passionate and dull as dirt. Think of them as role models for an aging society.

The United States is on the brink of a longevity revolution, according to the Centers for Disease Control and Prevention. The average American's life span has increased from nearly 55 in 1915 to almost 78. By 2030, the number of people aged 65 and older will have almost doubled and will make up nearly one-fifth of the population. We're growing older with the help of vaccinations, controls on infectious diseases, improvements in food safety, a decline in heart disease, antismoking campaigns, workplace safety, and better prenatal care. But it's not because we are exercising more. The

Getting Enough Exercise

According to the Centers for Disease Control and Prevention, moderate-intensity activities, the type needed in order to meet the agency's goal of 30 minutes of exercise five days a week, can be brisk walking, bicycling, vacuuming, gardening, or anything that causes a small increase in breathing rate. Adults can exercise harder and spend less time at it. For example, by doing 20 minutes of exercise three times a week, they still get the same health benefits. More difficult exercises include running, aerobics classes, and heavy yard work.

CDC says that men and women 18 and older need at least 30 minutes of physical activity five days a week.

Still, the consensus of experts is that half of adults who start an exercise regimen quit in six months or less. Only about 3 in 10 adults ages of 25 to 64 get enough leisure-time physical activity. After people reach 65, activity levels drop further. Nearly one-third of the U.S. adult population is obese.

"The reason for this ridiculously high dropout rate is that most exercise is not purposeful," said William Morgan, professor emeritus and sport psychologist at the University of Wisconsin–Madison. Older athletes, he said, find purpose in sweat. Morgan coined the term *exercise addiction* in 1979 for the small percentage of people who are so obsessed with working out that they get hooked on it. He believes a few older athletes have the affliction, but in most cases injuries take their toll first.

"I think those who are in sports and have been at it for a long time—especially the elite—probably do it because it's a part of their life," said David Costill, the founder of the Human Performance Laboratory at Ball State University. "It's just something they do, and their life isn't complete unless they do it." Costill has spent most of his life studying athletes, including older athletes. He was a collegiate swimmer but did not swim seriously again until he was 47. Two years later, he became a national champion in his age group. He described older athletes as "self-challengers—if it wasn't for masters swimming or running, they would create something that would be a challenge to them."

Many of those who return to a sport or get more serious about exercise do so after wandering for periods in a kinetic wilderness. When they come back, there is inevitably a period of transition. The body must adapt. Time must be carved out of the day. New skills must be learned or old skills grudgingly relearned. Many who aspire to return are shocked at how much they've lost.

When I started sprinting again, I looked for whatever I could find about middle-aged speedsters and quickly became a fan of masterstrack.com. There, men and women detail their struggles with injuries and their efforts to adapt workouts to their aging bodies. One day, a 50-something man named Taliq wrote about trying to run to catch the bus and missing it. In a moment of failure, he discovered how much of his former self was gone. He wanted to run fast again. "My goal is simply to be able to stride a quarter (mile) again to experience the joy of movement that only a runner knows when the mind stops and you are just into the flow," he wrote. "I've never run long enough or far enough to experience a second wind, so I don't have any illusions about being able to do it now. But for the sake of my health and peace of mind, I know I've got to compete again because it is what's missing from my life and, deep down, beneath all of my efforts to be realistic and humble, I still think that I can win a race against my peers."

Several people responded, including Ken Stone, a journalist from San Diego and the man behind the Web site. "I have an incredible amount of respect for older sprinters pursuing comebacks," he wrote. "I'm constantly battling a dilemma similar to yours: By what right should I expect to be a sprinter again after all of these years? My flippant answer: I'm an adult, and I can do whatever the hell I want to. My more nuanced answer is I'm an adult and I choose to live my childhood dream. The devil is in the details. You'll find out soon enough that sprinting in the late 50s is hellaciously demanding."

JAVELINS AT TWILIGHT

One night in 2001 at the National Masters Track & Field Championships in Baton Rouge, Louisiana, where I was competing in my first big national meet, I sat in the stands with Lynne Ingalls of Chicago. As we watched the races below us, javelins in an adjoining field propelled by old arms arced through the twilight, climbing higher and higher until gravity pulled them back to earth. Ingalls would be turning 59 the next day and she ruminated on a new stage in her life.

"You've gone to college," she said. "You have had your family. Your kids are married. And now it's back to taking care of yourself. I want to test my own limits and challenge myself personally. I don't think I have ever done that before. I was like so many of us who sat back and said I could do that, but never made the effort to find out—win, lose, or draw."

Until she sold a cleaning business she'd owned for 23 years, she often trained alone after work late at night. At a high school track in suburban Evanston, her workouts bordered on the surreal as she pushed herself to exhaustion, with motion detectors flicking on the lights as she moved around the oval. "That was either stupidity or passion," she said. "I like to call it passion. It was the best part of my day. I really looked forward to it. To me, running fast represents a sense of freedom, of flying. When you are out there on a track—and I am out there alone a lot—it is the freest feeling in the whole world."

When she returned home from Baton Rouge, she found a coach, started poring over technical journals, and enrolled in track clinics. Running was consuming more and more of her life, and eventually she became a coach for the University of Chicago Laboratory Schools' high school track team. The next summer, she would be part of a women's relay team that broke a world record.

Testing Yourself

The President's Challenge Adult Fitness Test (www.adultfitnesstest.org) is a Web site that gives you an idea of how you compare with someone your own age. You will be tested and scored for aerobic fitness, muscular strength and endurance, flexibility, and body composition. For example, for muscular strength if you are a 50-year-old male and can do 50 push-ups in a minute, you are in the 95th percentile; at 25 push-ups, you are in the 80th percentile. For aerobic fitness a 50-year-old woman who can run 1.5 miles in 12 minutes (an 8-minute mile) makes the 95th percentile; at 20 minutes her performance falls to the 30th percentile. You can test yourself periodically to see if you can improve your score.

There are the newcomers like Ingalls, and then there are the older athletes who have never left their sports. One of the first older sprinters I met was Stan Druckrey, a member of U.S. Masters Track and Field Hall of Fame. We both live in metropolitan Milwaukee, and one spring morning when he was 50, I joined him near his home for a workout. It was an interval day—a series of sprints to improve speed endurance that would be his hardest session of the week. With a few minutes of rest, we sprinted 500 meters, 400 meters, 300 meters, 200 meters, 100 meters, and finally 50 meters. As we rested, we talked occasionally. But mostly we listened to the birds and relished the blush of greenery around us. At each start, all we could hear was our breathing and the drum roll of our feet over the surface of the track. I tried to stay within a step or two of him, but the difference between me and a world-class masters athlete was clear. At the end of each interval, I would fall behind, while Druckrey's driving legs, the lightness of his feet, and his strong arm action seemed to push him effortlessly across the track.

Druckrey's specialty is the hurdles, and he made it to the Olympic Trials in 1972. His form is so good that he was once hired by an ad agency looking for a middle-aged runner to hurdle down a track in a Sansabelt blazer. At age 52, he went back to his alma mater to run against collegiate hurdlers. I asked him once, while we were having breakfast, how seriously he took the prospect of going up again men who were 30 years younger. Wasn't he doing it for fun? He glared at me. "Oh, no, no, no, no, no, no!" he said in a loud voice at a pancake house. "I don't put spikes on to say that I am going to run this for fun. That's a fun run. That's a three-mile run. This isn't fun. When there's a gun (several startled diners look up from their eggs) and people are watching, I'm racing. I came back to show these college kids what I can do."

TRAINING LIKE A PROFESSIONAL

Older athletes are able to tap into the countless number of advances made possible by the huge infusion of money into sports. In Baton Rouge, one of the men I ran against was Neville Hodge, then 45. He was bald and crow's-feet crinkled like river deltas around his eyes. He was the track coach at Morgan State University in Baltimore and a three-time Olympian for the United States Virgin Islands. He told me he videotaped his workouts so that he could look for flaws in his running. Afterward, he sat in an ice bath to reduce inflammation in his muscles. He thought such tools helped him break the world record that year for the 100-meter dash in our age group in a scary-fast 10.96 seconds. In the early 1900s, he would have been among the fastest sprinters in the world—regardless of age.

Even for those with much less talent, a cottage industry of fitness training has mushroomed to help older athletes. Technology also helps. A 60-year-old swimmer can glide through the water in the same drag-resistant swimsuits as Olympians. A weekend cyclist with an extra $7,000 or $8,000 can pedal models of carbon-fiber bicycles favored in the Tour de France. There are heart-rate monitors, body-fat calculators, and low-impact exercise equipment specifically designed to reduce the wear and tear on the body.

Baby boomers "are the first generation that never stopped exercising," said Dr. Nicholas DiNubile, an orthopedic surgeon who specializes in sports medicine and is a clinical assistant professor of the department of orthopaedic surgery at the Hospital of the University of Pennsylvania. In the late 1990s, he came up with a description for ailing jocks—he called it "boomeritis"—after he found himself treating a steady stream of adults who refused to temper their exercise as they got older. DiNubile likes to say that we've extended our life span, but we have not extended the warranty on our bodies. Muscles, bones, tendons, tissues, spinal disks all deteriorate with time. He counsels his clients to exercise regularly, to avoid overuse injuries by moderating or diversifying activities, and to get good rehabilitation after an injury. "Every time I'm in the office, I'm treating someone who's been injured in their effort to be fit," he said.

But the threat of injury isn't an excuse for life on the couch. The human body was made to be used. Today, swimmers in middle age are capable of turning in their fastest times ever. Men and women are building muscle mass in their 80s.

Weight training actually can make muscles younger, according to a 2007 study by the Buck Institute for Age Research in Novato, California. Researcher Simon Melov examined the mitochondrial function of muscle of men and women who were 65 and older and compared the results with those of men and women in their late teens and 20s. He took samples of muscle tissue before and after six months of resistance training and found that the old muscles had genetic characteristics similar to the muscles of the younger population.

When James Fries of Stanford University began a long-term study of runners in 1984, many scientists feared that the running boom would produce a flood of orthopedic injuries or cause permanent damage to its practitioners in old age. Fries, now a professor emeritus of medicine at Stanford, didn't think that would happen. He reasoned that keeping the body moving would extend longevity. Unquestionably, running can cause wear and tear. But it also helps muscles, ligaments, and bones become stronger, said Dr. Eliza Chakravarty of Stanford, a rheumatologist and one of the authors of the study, whose results were published in 2008. The study of 500 runners found that they had fewer disabilities, had a longer active life span, and were half as likely to die at an early age as a comparable group of nonrunners. "There are tremendous benefits to regular exercise," Chakravarty told me.

And it can be fun. When I began using spiked track shoes, it was like wearing glasses for the first time. Everything changed. I felt like I was running with bare feet and claws. Track meets were another thing. They scared the hell out of me. I was fit but by no means the fastest. But in workouts when I was brimming with energy, there were moments when I was swept up in the hallucinatory optimism of a sprinter's high: I was evading the tag; the ball was falling into my outstretched arms. It was the kinetic equivalent of standing in front of the mirror with the stereo cranked while strumming my air guitar. When I was finished with a workout, I would walk slowly around the track to cool down. It was my time for reflection. Ideas flowed in and out of my head like water through a tide pool.

Then there was the cold reality of the stopwatch. In Baton Rouge, I came in last in two races—the 100-meter and 200-meter dashes. A year's worth of work was over in less than a minute. In the 200, I was nipped at the finish line by Kelly Meares of Carl Junction, Missouri. We stood hunched over, gasping for breath and barely able to talk. "I thought you had me," he said. I said something like "Good race" and we shook hands. I walked away feeling angry at myself and embarrassed.

All the more so because the day before I had interviewed Floyd "Chunk" Simmons, a bronze medalist in the decathlon in the 1948 and 1952 Olympics. Simmons was there to throw the shot and the discus. He was suave and still handsome in his 70s. (He died in 2008 at the age of 84.) It was easy to see why he became a Hollywood actor and moved in the same circles as another aspiring actor, Clint Eastwood. "I know your game," he told me after my races. "You're one of those George Plimpton guys. You're here to experience it so you can write about it."

His comment stung because he didn't consider me on par with most of the others. But what he said was right: Not only did I bring my spikes, I brought notebooks and a tape recorder too. As much as I wanted to run fast, I wanted to explore the lives of the aging athletes. It was my last track meet, but sprinting was the springboard for this book.

I still train hard, but I've learned that variety is what keeps me going. I'm back to the old sports like running, cycling, swimming, and cross-country skiing; I still sprint; and I've added new things. At 50, I took up skateboarding. Last year, when I was 54, I had an old Peugeot my son found on the curb converted into a fixed-gear bike like those ridden by bicycle messengers.

Older athletes find things that suit them. They soldier on past the bad days when it all seems like drudgery. They find joy and meaning in pushing their bodies, and they live for those special fleeting moments when their powers seem limitless and everything seems possible.

A Note About Information Sources

All direct and indirect quotations are based on personal interviews, unless otherwise noted in the text or in references section of the book. All of the principal subjects I profiled in *Second Wind* were interviewed in person—either at sporting events, in their homes, or at other venues. In most cases, I also conducted numerous follow-up interviews by phone and e-mail.

The majority of event times, records, performances, and statistical information came from organizers of competitions, sport organizations, or their governing bodies. In a few instances, information came from the subjects themselves.

As background, I drew information from numerous sources: books, magazines, newspapers, scientific journals, government documents, film documentaries, television broadcasts, and Web sites.

Part I

Starting Out

It's never too late to find your inner athlete. Most people who start exercising, or try picking up a new sport, end up quitting. But it doesn't have to be this way. Some older athletes start after years of inactivity. Others come back from serious injuries. Athletes in middle age can sometimes duplicate what they did in their youth. This is especially true in swimming, where men and women are taking advantage of the latest improvements in training and technique. The key is that whatever activity you choose, it has to become a part of your life. Sweat is good.

1

From the Bench to the Bench Press

In the summer of 2006, I met Faith Ireland at her elegant club on the 75th floor of a Seattle skyscraper. The Columbia Tower Club affords sweeping views of the city, Puget Sound, and a snow-capped Mount Rainer in the distance. Ireland had recently retired from the Washington State Supreme Court, and when she greeted me, she glided across the room with the dignity of a robed justice.

We sipped ice water with lemon as our conversation touched a little on law and more on Ireland's lifelong quest for self-improvement, from her early struggles in the classroom, through an ambitious professional career, and then a most unexpected course: Ireland's venture into powerlifting.

She trains in the basement of a downtown office building, a no-frills gym where sweat and liniment mingle in the air with the sound of clanging iron. We met there later. She had changed into black shorts and a turquoise T-shirt with the words "USA Powerlifting." Sweat trickled down her forehead and over her makeup. A thick leather belt was cinched around her waist. She stood on a hard rubber mat in front of a metal bar holding 255 pounds (102 kg). She repeated to herself, "Calm, strong, and powerful." It is her mantra. "People think of powerlifting as 'You see heavy stuff, you pick up heavy stuff,'" she once told me. "But it's very technical and you have to have your head in the right place."

She was practicing her deadlifts, which her barrel-chested coach, Todd Christensen, described as the "truest test of overall strength—it's the lift that involves the most muscle fibers in the body." Ireland took hold of the bar with an alternating overhand and underhand grip, which exposed the manicured fingernails on her left hand. She took a deep breath. Ireland, who at the time was 63 years old (she was born in 1942), lifted the bar until she had straightened her back and brought the weight to her midthighs. She grimaced as she held it aloft. It was her third such lift in a row. Christensen signaled and she brought the bar down.

"That's great, girl!" Christensen said. "Nice lift."

Ireland nodded and swaggered away.

Powerlifting consists of the deadlift, the squat, and the bench press. The sport is considered one of the ultimate tests of pure strength; in fact, it is often powerlifters (or former powerlifters) who participate in strongman competitions, engaging in tests of superhuman strength—like strapping themselves in a harness and pulling jetliners over tarmacs. In contrast to bodybuilders, who are virtually naked in competition, powerlifters are often wrapped in suits of Lycra and Kevlar to provide extra support. The atmosphere of a gym can seem indelicate if not downright intimidating. With so much exertion, it is not uncommon to hear the sound of passing gas. "We're not always ladylike," Ireland told me with a smile. Lifts can include raucous and elaborate psyche-up rituals. And when the lift is successful, the grimace and bulging eyes can be a portrait of ecstatic physical pleasure. In practice at Ireland's gym, fellow lifters are apt to pause and shout encouragement when one of them is working on a big lift. After an especially impressive set, Christensen would say admiringly, "Somebody's getting stronger!"

Powerlifting builds muscle mass, and some lifters are known to craft huge, cartoonish physiques—even in Ireland's federation, USA Powerlifting, where at least 10 percent of competitors at meets are drug tested and subject to random testing. But even though Ireland has gotten stronger since she began lifting in 1999, weightlifting has been the key factor in her losing weight. She weighed a doughy 165 pounds (75 kg) when she started. At 5-foot-3 (160 cm), she dropped to as low as 124 pounds (56 kg) and now competes in the 132-pound (60 kg) weight class. Her diet is better and lifting has stoked her metabolism. Workouts can last two hours or more, three nights a week. Active muscle tissue needs more energy than fat—even if it's resting on the couch. Running or another exercise would have made Ireland fit, but she opted for weights.

"Why screw with it?" she said. "It's the fountain of youth. I mean, I'm more healthy than when I was 42. People tell me that all of the time—and I'm not even a justice any more."

Ireland is a four-time national age-group champion powerlifter—in 2002, 2004, 2007, and 2008. At her weight class, she holds all of the American records in the 65 to 69 age group. In an international meet in the Czech Republic in 2003, she won a bronze medal in the bench press. In India in 2004, she won a silver medal, even though she was lumped in with women in her weight class who were as young as 50.

As Ireland has grown older, she has lifted more weight. In 2002, at the national championships in Chicago, she lifted a combined weight of 539 pounds (244 kg). In 2007 in Baton Rouge at the women's nationals, she lifted a combined 641.3 pounds (291 kg)—102 pounds more. Then, at the International Powerlifting Federation world meet in Palm Springs, California, in October 2008, Ireland, at age 66, had lifts totaling 654.5 pounds. It was a remarkable display of strength for someone her age. Ireland's bench press of 137.5 pounds (61 kg) in Palm Springs meant she can bench more than her own weight—a common test of superior upper body strength.

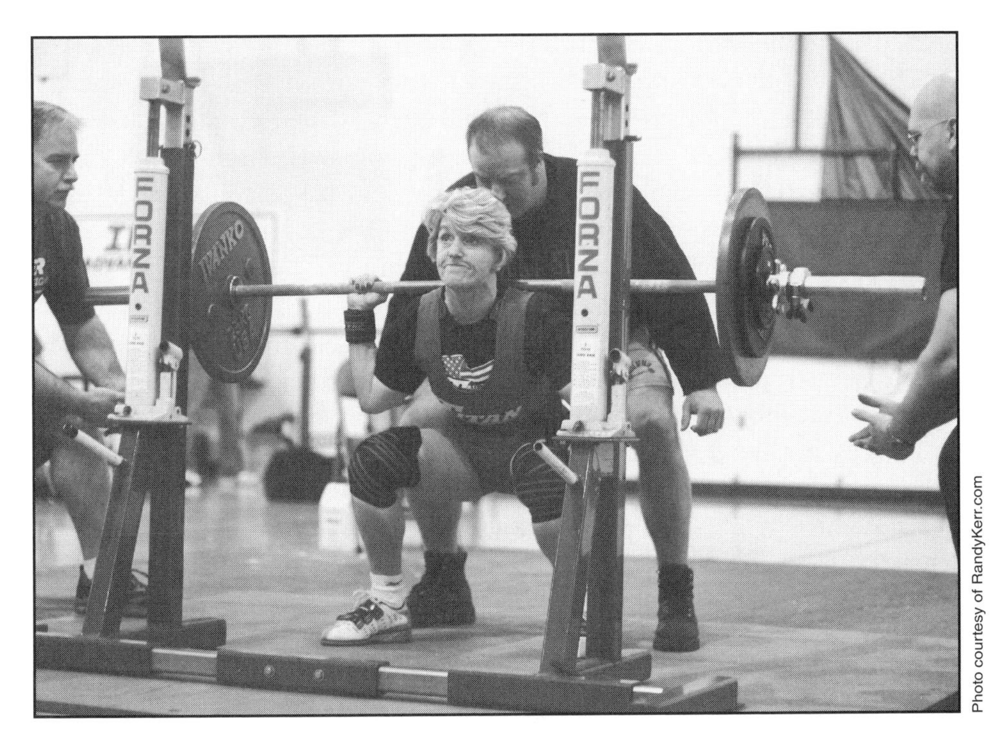

Photo courtesy of RandyKerr.com

Faith Ireland competes at the second annual Fife Power Company Powerlifting.

"Faith has not plateaued," Christensen told me when we met in his gym, Seattle Strength and Power, before Ireland and his other clients arrived. "I don't think it's a matter of age—it's how long you have been in the sport." What Christensen meant is that men and women can become stronger as they age. However, they won't improve if they have been lifting as long and as intensively as he has. Christensen was 45 years old when we met in 2006. He was 5-foot-11 and weighed 242 pounds (180 cm, 110 kg). He could bench 550 pounds (249 kg) and held world records for his age group in the bench press. But he had peaked as a powerlifter because he had been lifting weights since he was a teenager. Ireland, meanwhile, took up powerlifting at 57.

"Faith started, what, six, seven years ago?" he said. "She might not peak until she is 70." Indeed, weight training can cushion what age can take away. A prevalent view is that most people peak at 25, followed by a slow physical spiral. After 40, the average person loses one-third to one-half pound of muscle a year. Usually, fat replaces muscle. But numerous studies have shown that men and women are capable of increasing muscle mass into their 80s. Weight training increases metabolism, fights osteoporosis, lowers blood pressure, and can help alleviate back pain.

Ireland, in fact, started lifting for the same reason many middle-aged people swear off any kind of weight training: She had a bad back. In 1983, she was appointed to fill a vacancy in King County Superior Court, which includes Seattle. It was a frenetic time for judges, she said, because the court system was not keeping up with the region's population growth. "For the next year it was a real roller-coaster ride," she said. She had to run for a full term. While campaigning, she was rear-ended in a hit-and-run accident and badly injured her back. Two weeks later, she became pregnant. She was 40 years old. The pregnancy was welcome news for Ireland and her husband. But it limited her ability to treat her back pain. Then, less than four weeks before the due date, the baby was stillborn.

The crash caused permanent damage to Ireland's neck and lower back and produced both sciatic pain and pounding headaches at the base of her skull. An arbitration panel eventually awarded her $182,833. When we met at her club, she described the sciatica as a "hot poker in the right buttocks." Numbness and pain radiated down her right leg. Her shoulders felt as if she were carrying a steel girder on them.

She tried Advil, light weights, water aerobics, physical therapy, and biofeedback. She went to a psychiatrist for grief counseling after losing the baby. As a result of the pregnancy, she gained 30 pounds.

Working Through the Pain

"I really do believe there are times when you need to work through the pain," said Dr. Nicholas DiNubile, an orthopedic surgeon who specializes in sports medicine. Exercise, he said, is a "powerful medication, a powerful stimulus. But generally, just to blow through the pain is not good advice."

DiNubile, who is a consultant to the Philadelphia 76ers and the author of *Framework: Your 7-Step Program for Healthy Muscles, Bones, and Joints*, can't speak directly to Ireland's case. But he noted that exercise regimens that involve stretching and core work, for example, can lay the groundwork for heavier workouts that come later.

Then in 1995 while presiding over a personal-injury case, a potential juror said he had once suffered back pain but cured himself by lifting weights. Ireland had heard this before, but what he said next intrigued her. "He said that he overcame his back injury by *ignoring* his doctor's advice to work out just to the point of pain," she said. "Instead, he worked *through* the pain. I thought that sounded very interesting and I decided that I was going to try that."

Ireland went back to a health club and began using big rubber balls, elastic bands, and three-pound weights. She was 55 years old—an ailing middle-aged woman, surrounded by muscle and mirrors. "I felt old, tired, and fat," she recalled in a speech in 2004 at the Washington State Senior Games. "Oh, yes, and I had a healthy dose of self-pity."

It hurt to lift. But gradually she began to feel better and was enjoying the aftereffects of a good workout. By 1997—2 years after lifting weights and after living with the effects of the car accident for 15 years—she was pain free.

A BIG LIFT

Ireland started powerlifting by accident. Her personal trainer had been Willie Austin, a former cornerback at the University of Washington and a former world powerlifting champion. One day, Austin had an appointment with another woman who was getting ready for a powerlifting competition. He asked Ireland to join them, and when they were finished, he suggested she enter the meet too.

"It was kind of a natural progression for her," said Paula Houston, who trains at Seattle Strength and Power. Houston has been a world champion in her 40s and was a world champion in open competition when she was younger. "Faith was getting stronger than she thought she could get," Houston said. "And when she saw all of us crazy powerlifters out there, she didn't know if she should really be there, so she just went along."

Powerlifting also appealed to Ireland's attraction to the limelight. Houston told me that Ireland is the only powerlifter she's seen who smiles before a lift. "I don't know if she realizes this, when she gets up on the squat platform, she gives the judges a big old smile before she lifts: 'I'm on stage. I'm ready for my close-up!'"

Ireland was elected to a six-year term on the Washington State Supreme Court in 1999. Not long after she joined the court, a Seattle columnist wrote that Ireland had won a local powerlifting competition. Another reporter called and wanted to write a longer story on the bench-pressing justice.

"Then I thought to myself, 'Was this a good thing, or not a good thing, for a supreme court justice to be doing, in the eyes of the public?'" she said. She concluded that if it got other people to exercise, or if it prompted others with back problems to lift weights and get healthy again, she should be talking about it.

Ireland decided not to run for a second term on the court. She was eager to reclaim her private life and had no appetite for spending a year campaigning across Washington. She took off six weeks to ski and attend a downhill ski camp in Sun Valley, Idaho, and then went back to work as a mediator and consultant. One of her first projects was to help an organization fight a group that was opposed to fluoridating the public water supply in Skagit County, Washington. She also served as vice chair of a panel looking into management practices of the King County Sheriff's Department.

"Faith is very motivated," Christensen said. "If she is going to do something, she is going to do it at the top level. It's like that with anything in her life."

When I visited the gym for the first time in 2004, a muscle-bound man 20 years younger than Ireland was struggling with his squat. Christensen told him to watch Ireland's technique. She seldom makes the same mistake twice.

Ireland was one of only two women in her 1969 law school class at Willamette University College of Law. She later received a master's degree in taxation. Before she was elected to Washington's high court, she served 15 years as a superior court judge.

But Ireland has had her share of setbacks and struggled with feelings of inadequacy. She was perplexed by math and science, and after a test in eighth grade her advisor recommended she pursue options other than college. She ran into the restroom and cried. Eventually, she came to see that moment as a gift. Even though the assessment was painful, she knew she was better than that. "Never believe someone who tells you that you can't do something," she told community college graduates in a commencement speech in 2000. But even when she did excel, "there was always the seed of doubt," she told me. In hindsight, she believes she suffered from imposter syndrome, which often afflicts high achievers who feel the urge to sabotage themselves. "You are waiting to be discovered to be the fraud that you think you are," she said.

At the University of Washington in 1965, she got pregnant. "I wanted to go kill myself," she told me. "I wanted to jump off the Aurora Bridge rather than go home and tell my parents that I was pregnant. Times were very different back then. I was sure they would disown me."

On her way to the bridge, she stopped at her church. It was locked. She went to a pay phone and called the church, hoping someone was inside. The call was routed to her minister, who came with his wife and counseled her. She didn't think her parents would be supportive, but they were. Then she made the hardest decision in her life and gave the baby up for adoption. In 1997, she reunited with her daughter, who is an artist living in New York. Ireland is now a grandmother.

Ireland, by her own description, is a "growth-group junkie," and her conversations are peppered with the language of self-improvement. "That's how I got to where I am in life—going though self-talk, having goals, visualizations that go with those goals, and affirmation to help me get through the tough times," she said.

How to Change Your Life

Powerlifting transformed Faith Ireland's life. Looking back, she recognizes how it happened. The discipline required for improvement in lifting weights was already deeply ingrained in her. One of the lessons instilled when she was growing up was to, in her words, "work hard and skillfully and never give up." When she speaks to groups, Ireland tells people to ask themselves what their most deeply held and most cherished values are. Usually it involves an important lesson that was learned. Then she asks whether they are living by those values. Living by those values makes people free, authentic, and fulfilled.

At the center of her belief system is the notion that "you can change your life by changing your thinking," she said. "It's never too late; you're never too busy." She has adopted this same mind-set with weightlifting. "You don't allow any thoughts of fear into your mind," she said. "Negative self-talk is always there at the ready. If someone starts talking about injuries, I get up and walk away." Ireland told me she sometimes psyches herself up for a big lift by imagining she is at a world championship and standing at the podium draped with an American flag and wearing a gold medal around her neck.

"Faith," Houston told me, "has been a wonderful mentor."

THE POWER OF NOW

When Houston (born in 1961) and I met in 2006 at the neighborhood YMCA she runs in Seattle, she was 45 years old. She has a master's degree in health administration and had long been a dominant force in powerlifting. But at one stage in her career, she thought she needed to be more entrepreneurial and leverage her expertise in strength and fitness to become a personal trainer. Ireland was one of her clients.

Houston smiled. "Hated it, *hated it*," she said. "When I was trying to run my business, and it wasn't going so well, I would come in and Faith could see through that in a second. She could tell the energy wasn't there."

Ireland gave Houston a book, *The Power of Now: A Guide to Spiritual Enlightenment*, by Eckhart Tolle, who, in Houston's words, urges people to "stop worrying about all of the stuff that goes on around you. To change, just take small steps to get there. Stay in the now, stay in the present, and know that everything is going to be OK."

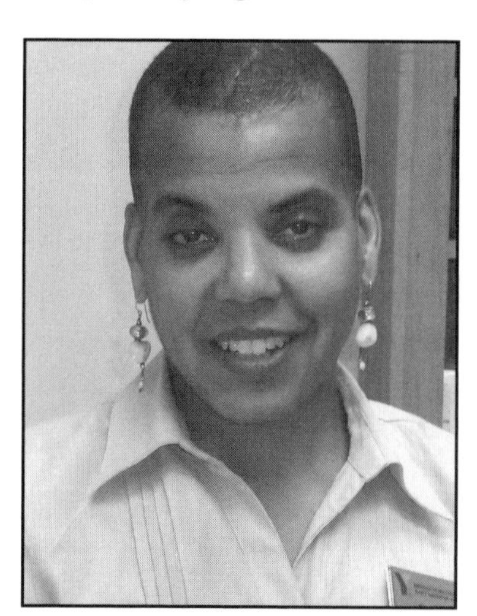

Faith Ireland's fellow powerlifter Paula Houston.

"That book saved my life—saved my sanity," Houston said.

Powerlifting "has kept me grounded," she said. "Now, because I have won a lot of championships—and don't get me wrong; it's still all about the winning—it's become part of my spiritual practice. It's what really keeps me centered. If something crazy is going on at work, I say to myself, 'You have two more hours and you're going to be working out and you can forget all of this,'" Houston said.

The next day at the gym, Houston was warming up by doing yoga. Ireland jumped rope and used 10- and 12-pound weights before starting her workout. She stood periodically next to a fan because of the effects of hot flashes. After she left the court, she went off hormone-replacement therapy, and like clockwork the hot flashes appeared every hour and a half. At night in bed to take her mind off the discomfort, she sometimes practices lifting an imaginary barbell.

The group that afternoon also included Terry Lee, 51, an IT manager who spends free time restoring antique linens, and Jill Arnow, 46, a studio artist. Like Houston and Ireland, they are national age-group powerlifting champions.

As of June 2008, Christensen's athletes had won seven International Powerlifting Federation championships, 23 USA Powerlifting championships, 25 World Association of Benchers and Deadlifters world championships, and more than 100 state championships. They had set 24 USAPL national records and more than 100 state records.

Seattle Strength and Power is located in a long, narrow subterranean room in downtown Seattle. On one of my visits, a diversity of music, including classic rock and hip-hop, poured from a pair of speakers. There is a small reception area and a locker room in the front. A single aisle separates a pair of weightlifting benches, five squat racks, and an assortment of wooden platforms covered with rubber lifting mats for deadlifts. Like heavy poker chips, weight plates are stacked everywhere. In the back of the room, Christensen keeps four huge tires, the largest weighing 1,000 pounds (454 kg), that lifters practice flipping for strongman contests. A dozen atlas lifting stones—100 to 360 pounds (45 to 163 kg)—lie on the floor. A German shorthaired pointer panhandled for attention.

Arnow's father had died recently and she got hugs from the others. At one of the squat racks, Terry Lee used an unorthodox style in which she leaned forward with the weight and then threw back her shoulders to compensate for two discs that had been removed in her back. Arnow and another lifter, Sharee Olson, 65, both have recovered from thyroid cancer. Another lifter was a recovering alcoholic. A man in his 30s was on kidney dialysis.

Ireland called the group a "collaboration of misfits"—a term of endearment. "A lot of us have some kind of limitation and we're pressing past that," she said.

When Ireland was on the court, she trained with Christensen twice a week and lifted a third day at another gym with her husband, Chuck Norem, who lifts to stay in shape for an age-group baseball league he plays

A Word From the Experts

Wayne L. Westcott and Thomas R. Baechle, coauthors of the 2007 book *Strength Training Past 50*, offer safety advice for older athletes looking to improve their strength without injury:

Use a spotter when performing the squat, bench press, and incline press. A failed repetition can result in serious injury. A competent spotter should stand behind the lifter ready to lift the bar during the bench or incline or to help the lifter return to a standing, upright position during the squat. Strength training after age 50 will aid athletic performance and aid in the management and prevention of arthritis, diabetes, and osteoporosis.

in. On days when she was in Olympia, the state capital, she would drive 60 miles back to Seattle for her workout. There were times, she admitted, when she was thinking more about torts than lifts. But inevitably, weightlifting leaves her "much more centered and focused and calm," she said.

Now she is working with Christensen three days a week. Between lifts, Ireland took notes about making improvements. One of her entries said, "Knees dropping in. Need to think. Need to think about pushing knees to the side—not the front." She relies on Christensen to guide her though the day's regimen. "Frankly, I don't pay much attention," she said. "I just do what he tells me to do. I don't try to second-guess him."

Christensen keeps a written plan on each of his clients. But as he moved among the women and their respective lifts, he seemed to have it all in his head. He uses a six- to eight-week cycle, aiming to get a maximum lift at the end of the cycle. Rather than have them try to lift the most they can at each session, he aims for something a little less. For example, on one visit, he told me he wanted his lifters to reach 80 percent of their maximum weight in five lifts—and have them do three sets.

Training middle-aged women has its advantages: "They listen to their bodies better," he said.

Ireland doesn't believe lifting has cured her back problems, but it's been her best protection against further injury. "I know that if I were out of the gym for four weeks, I would start to get sciatic pain again," she said. She has never been injured since she took it up, but she has had setbacks ("bombing out," as she calls it) by not making a lift at a meet once in a while.

Later Ireland sent me an e-mail about a performance in Seattle that was both "terrific" and "awful," because she made only three of nine lifts. The gym was stifling and her arms swelled up as she struggled to wedge her torso into a specially designed shirt made of supportive synthetic material that is intended to improve a lifter's performance. Getting the right fit, and matching it to the strength of a lifter, is a mix of art and science. Ireland still managed to set a new American record, however, in the squat. Afterward some of the lifters went to her house, drank beer, ate pizza, and watched the moon rise over Lake Washington.

By the end of her e-mail, she seemed more upbeat about how the meet went. "Two rounds of ice packs on my back and quads and I feel really good again today!" she wrote. "There is something about doing this stuff that makes you think you can do anything."

Ireland often wins her age group because in some tournaments there is little competition—the universe of 60-something female powerlifters is small. "At first when I started doing this, it didn't feel like winning," she told me when we first met at her club. "But I came to appreciate the fact that, yeah, I really had to make these lifts in the first place. And then I started breaking records, and that made me feel better."

Ireland said older athletes have to be willing to deal with the ups and downs of their sport. "That's where a lot of people fall out," she said. "They're willing to do it as long as they get all of the goodies. But once they get the setbacks, they don't want to start over. That's where the mental toughness that comes with maturity can be a real advantage."

2

The Comeback

Like getting out of debt, the act of returning to a sport can be an arduous journey. Every weekend, legions of middle-aged men and woman have visions of once again becoming athletes. But most people in middle age who pick up a sport or start exercising soon give up. The comeback is a minefield of setbacks and wrong turns. It's too hard. It takes time. The payoff isn't quick. And the threat of injury is a grim reality.

After decades of being away from their games, I met three men who came back and become the best in their age groups. John Sorce and Thomas Weisel had remained physically active as adults. But Gerald Vaughn had done little since college. Sorce, a speed skater, and Weisel, a cyclist, desperately wanted to become champions. They knew what they wanted and they methodically put themselves in a position to reach their goals. Vaughn is a bear of a man, a shot putter, who has grown stronger as he has become older. He, too, is driven to break records—to toss a metal ball farther than any man ever in his 70s. But early on, it was grief that pushed him into the gym.

JOHN SORCE: FIRE ON ICE

John Sorce (born in 1933) hadn't been on the ice in 47 years, and as he watched the skaters glide around the oval, he wondered whether he could ever race like that again. He was 65. He had once been a promising skater. At 17, even though he had slipped in one race and fallen in two others, he had come in second in a national speed skating championship. "That bugged me," he said. "It's bugged me all of my life."

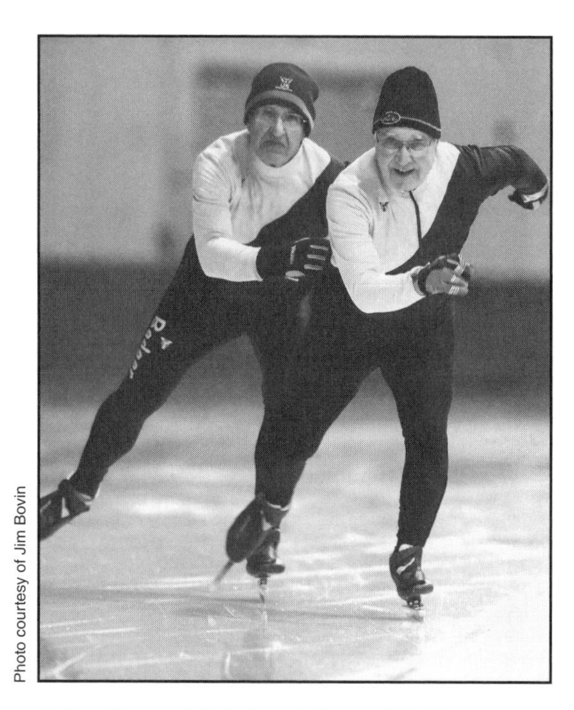

Photo courtesy of Jim Bovin

John Sorce (right) training with Vern Kappes.

Now years later, the skaters he was watching weren't kids. They were his age, and seeing them brought back a flood of memories—the old ice rink, racing on the weekend, and trying to make the 1952 Olympic Trials but coming up short. He played baseball in college, he taught dancing, and there were all those years of playing golf. But as he watched the men skate, his old sport seemed so intoxicating. The ice glistened like liquid plastic. The long, graceful strides of the skaters cut the surface like sharp knives. After each race, they sat down, laughed, and kibitzed. Sorce—who pronounces his name "source"—was certain that years ago he had beaten a bunch of them.

The next day, he was on the starting line. An old friend had encouraged him to go home and get his skates. A lot had changed. There was no biting wind at the Pettit National Ice Center in West Allis, Wisconsin, a suburb of Milwaukee. The 400-meter rink is one of only three covered ovals in North America. The skates the men wore were a combination of graphite, leather, and sharp steel—some costing as much as $2,000. Sorce was wearing a pair of his frayed leather Planerts from the 1940s. Most of the others had been training and racing all season long—for years, even decades. He would be cramming for an ancient history exam.

The gun fired. "In your mind you think that you're probably 10 times better than you are," he recalled. "I was shocked that I was so uncompetitive. I couldn't keep up. I never dreamed that I wouldn't be in the thick of things." Nervous, and out of skating shape, he fell in one race and finished 50 yards behind the leaders in another.

With his crash-and-burn approach, Sorce faced a cold reality: Had strapping on the skates been a mere dalliance? Or was there something else going on—something so captivating that he had to pursue it?

Golf had been John Sorce's game when he lived in Arizona in the winter during the early years of his retirement. He would return to Wisconsin in the summer. The more time he spent in the North, the more he wanted to come back for good. His wife wanted to stay in Tucson. "You go to the hardware store, the dry cleaners," he said. "Where are we going to eat tonight? The cocktail hour was the most important thing. I didn't fit in."

He divorced and moved back home to Janesville. He got back into the real estate business and began developing residential lots on 140 acres he owned on the Rock River. He started clearing brush and restoring land to native prairie. In the winter, he took up cross-country skiing.

In the summer of 1997, he spotted Vern Kappes at a golf tournament in Janesville. They hadn't seen each other in almost 40 years. Kappes, who is the same age as Sorce, has spent most of his life living a few miles from the Pettit National Ice Center and its outdoor predecessor, where the two of them had skated as kids. Back then, Sorce beat Kappes most of the time. He knew if he got back into the sport, he wanted to be an age-group champion like Kappes. He'd want to beat his old friend. "It was a goal to get back to that level," he said.

That fall had marked his ignominious return. Kappes, who had finished far ahead, hadn't missed a season since 1939. Sorce went to work. He bought a book on speed skating that helped him work on conditioning and technique. He also had to adjust to a technological innovation called the clap skate—a hinged mechanism that allows the back of the blade to break away from the boot and stay on the ice longer.

During fall and winter, he would get up at seven o'clock, eat two English muffins with peanut butter and jelly, and drive an hour and 15 minutes three days a week to West Allis to train. He would skate with several clubs. If it was a heavy workout with younger skaters, "you were hyperventilating all the way back to Janesville," he said. Other times, he trained with Kappes and worked on racing strategy. "He didn't hold back," Sorce said. "He helped me improve my technique. We got to be very competitive, but it was good." Sorce even hired his own coaches. One year he skated with Luke Langer, an Olympic hopeful. Langer needed money and Sorce needed the help. "One day he told me he didn't have enough money to pay for gas and I said, 'For crying out loud, why don't you coach me?' It was my way of helping." Another year, he worked with four-time Olympian Nancy Swider-Peltz. In the winter of 2003-4, he hired another former Olympian, David Cruikshank, husband of gold medalist Bonnie Blair. On training days, he'd be away from home for five hours.

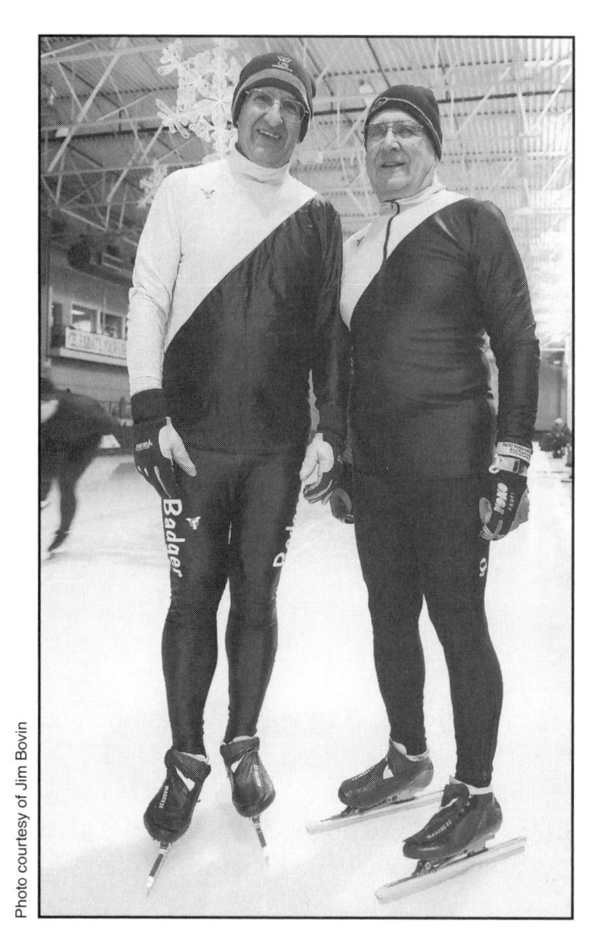

Photo courtesy of Jim Bovin

Vern Kappes (left) with John Sorce in 2007. Kappes has competed every year since he began skating in 1939.

One morning in February 2004, Sorce was practicing alone at the Pettit. He was wearing black tights, a striped sweater, and a muffler that he pulled up over his mouth. On a bench next to the ice was his gym bag with the words "Skate Now, Work Later." He usually warmed up by stretching, jogging around the oval, and skating two miles, "maybe testing yourself, going as hard as you can the last two laps," he told me. Then it was on to a series of intervals, skating distances from 200 to 1,600 meters at nearly top speed. He also worked on his start.

All of his training had paid off. His mechanics had become smoother since the last time I had watched him skate two years earlier. His arms and legs worked more in unison. He skated lower and could jackknife his body into a 90-degree crouch that let him drive his legs harder. He had the look of the graceful skater he had wanted to be. He had skated for more than an hour and when he was done, his eyes sparkled.

How did he feel?

"Happier," he said. There was a spring in his step. At 5-foot-7 (170 cm) and 167 pounds (76 kg), he weighed about 10 pounds more than when he played baseball at the University of Wisconsin–Madison. "During most of my life, it was business and career," he said. "You're not in condition. You go to cocktail parties. You're not eating the right foods. My hours are more regular now. I'll indulge in a glass of wine. But I am much more health conscious."

It took Sorce five years to get back into top form. "It's like golf," he said. "Every year when you start, you have no idea where the club head is when you bring it back. You're starting all over again."

Kappes agreed: "Speed skating is a physical sport—it's a power sport. You have to stay in shape. If you're not, you know it the first time you go to the line. It kept me from drinking and smoking and letting my body get out of shape."

In the United States, masters skate pack style, meaning they line up without the protection of their respective lanes. At the start, their clap skates sound like ponies galloping over cobblestones. The clamor fades as they gain speed and each stroke grows longer. Like distance runners in a track meet, they jostle for position and adjust to the ebb and flow of the race.

"In pack style you know where you are right away," Kappes said. "You know who you've got to beat and who's beating you."

Sorce admitted he gets uptight before a race. At a meet I attended, he nervously eyed a beefy, ungainly man he would be skating with and worried he'd box him out at a turn. "The first day of a big race is the worst," he told me. Vern always says to me, 'John, just consider it a regular day, a training session.' But it doesn't work out that way."

Kappes thinks his friend takes racing too seriously. "For him, being he took all of those years off, he gets butterflies," he said. "I just can't anymore. To me it's just another day of skating. I don't have any trouble sleeping the night before a race. He can't sleep."

At the 2004 National Long Track Championships in West Allis, Sorce won the first two races for the 70-to-79 age group, and the next day, Kappes won the next two. The overall standings are won by the number of points skaters earn in five races ranging from 500 to 3,000 meters.

The national champion would be decided in the final race—the 3,000 meters. The number of older speed skaters isn't big, and at the nationals, the 60- and 70-year-old age brackets were skating together. Kappes was leading his age group, drafting behind a Maryland skater in his 60s.

"Vern is a good sprinter," Sorce said. "But he's different from me. I got quick feet. He's all power. One hundred yards, 200 yards—he's coming—300 yards and he'll move around the corner well. He'll finish well with that 200 pounds of his. When he's moving like that, it's hard to beat him."

Kappes knew that he wanted to press the pace and stick with the Maryland skater as long as he could. "I made the decision from the start that I was going to chase this guy," he said. "The guy set a very fast pace and I wanted to see if I could extend myself that long." He knew Sorce would draft behind him, but he hoped as the pace quickened toward the finish, he could stay ahead.

Kappes led the whole race. Then in the final three meters, Sorce passed him. "I honestly didn't know if I would catch him," Sorce said. "I worked for five years to beat him."

Sorce broke the national record for his age group in the 3,000 when he crossed the line at 5:03.73. At the age of 71, he had finally won a national long-track title.

Adapted, by permission, from K. Stone, 2001, "Conquering our minds is biggest hurdle." Article is no longer available online at www.masterstrack.com.

Perspectives on Aging and Athleticism

James Lofton, NFL Hall of Fame, now a sprinter and long jumper

"I got football out of my system," he said. "A lot of guys who were in the league are too banged up to do track—or they just don't care. A lot of former athletes get into the business world and they love to compete there. I just always kept working out." He now competes in masters track events. "Winning is a minor part of it," he said. "For me, track and field is pure enjoyment."

Courtland Gray, Masters Track & Field Hall of Fame

He was a hurdler at Navy and returned to the sport at age 49. Many who reached the pinnacle of their sport think that doing anything less is trivial. "It was so tough to get to that level that when it's over, it's like school: You don't want to go back," he said. In fact, when he runs an exceptional race, "it's a good feeling—but I expect to run fast, and I expect to get over the hurdles without screwing up." He gets a greater thrill out of a great shot on the golf course or on the tennis court. "Because I don't expect to stick it on the green or hit that perfect ace," he said.

Todd Christensen, former NFL all-pro tight end, now competes in track

After retirement from football, he continued to lift weights and run six days a week. Then, he took up the multievent pentathlon and decathlon in his 40s. At a track meet, he pulled up his T-shirt and modeled a set of rippling six-pack abs. Much of his motivation for working out stems from a longstanding fear of getting fat. At the age of 12, he saw former NFL great Paul Hornung broadcasting a football game on TV. "He was 250 pounds," Christensen said. "His belly was out to here. That was the Golden Boy. And I remember thinking to myself at the time, 'Man, I don't want to look like that.'"

THOMAS WEISEL: MASTER OF THE UNIVERSE

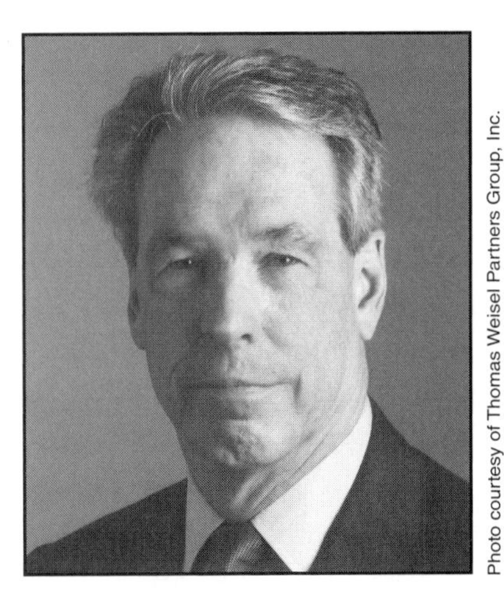
Photo courtesy of Thomas Weisel Partners Group, Inc.

Thomas Weisel.

Like John Sorce, Thomas Weisel (born in 1941) had also been a skater in Milwaukee. As a teen, he had been a national champion and had a good chance of making the 1960 Olympic team. In the fall of 1959, he left home to attend Stanford University, convinced that he could exercise and study before taking off the winter quarter to get back into skating shape and make the team. "I stupidly decided to go to Stanford for a quarter and couldn't train," Weisel told me in his office in downtown San Francisco. Many of the skaters had been training all fall and winter. At the trials that winter, Weisel lost out. It hurt even more because a skater he had beaten would medal at Squaw Valley. "I think as a result of that I'm pretty much of a frustrated athlete," he said.

After graduating from Stanford, Weisel went to Harvard for an MBA and has had a successful career in finance. He helped start Montgomery Securities and is the founder of Thomas Weisel Partners, a merchant bank.

Even though he failed to make the Olympic team, he kept his hand in athletics. He raced in downhill skiing. He took up long-distance running. He also got involved in multisport competitions among West Coast financiers called the Summer Rally Olympic Games. At age 40 he could still run a 50.6-second quarter mile.

When we met in 2001, a framed yellow jersey from Lance Armstrong and the Tour de France was displayed prominently on the wall. Aside from Armstrong, there are few people more responsible for helping to fuel the growth of American cycling than Weisel. At Montgomery Securities, Weisel formed a sports division to finance a bicycling team and he found himself rubbing shoulders with the elite of American cycling. He bankrolled Armstrong after Armstrong's French team, Cofidis, dropped him after he was diagnosed with testicular cancer. Weisel also brought together wealthy friends to bail out the financially ailing USA Cycling, the national governing body of the sport.

Cycling and speed skating have always had a symbiotic relationship. Skaters traditionally have cycled in the summer to stay in shape, and so did a young Weisel, often riding on a banked velodrome at a park a few miles from his home.

Skiing had battered his knees, so in his 40s, Weisel found himself gravitating to cycling again. But this was the 1980s—before Armstrong's seven Tour de France victories that helped spur the popularity in the sport.

Weisel has a reputation for being fiercely competitive in business—and he approached cycling in the same way. He wasn't content to pedal with poseurs on weekends. "You've got to compete if you want to see what you are made of," he said in his 2003 biography, written with Richard Brandt, *Capital Instincts: Life as an Entrepreneur, Financier, and Athlete*. "If you don't risk anything, you don't accomplish anything."

Like other successful middle-aged athletes, Weisel had the fire and requisite skills. In his weight room at home, he taped a picture on the wall of his archrival for motivation. But what separated Weisel from virtually anyone else was his ability to tap the best coaching in the country. Just as in finance, he wanted an edge—something that only the best know-how would provide. He sought out Eddie Borysewicz, a native of Poland who coached the 1980 and 1984 U.S. Olympic teams. "I said, 'Eddie, I know how to run on a track but I don't know how to train on a bicycle,'" Weisel told me. "'Can we get together? Can we train together?'"

Weisel hired "Eddie B" as his coach in 1985. He also attended Borysewicz's camps, sometimes jetting down to San Diego in his own plane after work to train with the maestro and some of the top riders in the country. The financial markets were slow in the late 1980s, so Weisel reasoned that he could commit more time to the sport than at any other time in his adult life. It took him several years to pull it all together: strength and endurance training, improving his technique, and honing racing strategies to attack and counterattack.

Weisel wasn't a long-distance specialist like Armstrong. He specialized in short races—criteriums and cat-and-mouse races on the velodrome where riders shadow each other for position before making a mad dash to the finish. He won national and world championships, including the kilo (an all-out sprint against the clock for 1 kilometer) in the World Masters Championships in 1991 at the age of 50.

"I treated myself as if I were an Olympic athlete," he said. "It was fun to see if I could accomplish in a different sport something that I couldn't get when I was 17 years old. It is a pretty myopic life. At the time I was not married. My three older kids were well on their way, so I didn't have to spend as much time with them. It was a perfect time to do it."

Still, he fretted over finding the right balance between work and cycling and staying in peak condition and not burning out. "The one thing that was really frustrating is that every time that I turned it up, in terms of conditioning, I would get sick," he said. "That would really frustrate me.

Then you'd have to quit for two weeks and get your body back and go at it again. I don't know if age had anything to do with it, but it's how my body reacted to it. When I would go 200 to 300 miles a week, man, I would pay for it. I must say that I would never do it again to get to that level of excellence."

GERALD VAUGHN: MOURNING A LOSS

Gerald Vaughn's wife of 40 years was dying of cancer. He would come home from work and take care of her. If he wasn't with her, he'd mope around the house. Maybe, she told him, he should get some exercise. Maybe he ought to try tossing his old shot around. Vaughn (born in 1935) found an old 12-pounder from high school and started throwing it into a backyard garden. It was the first time he had thrown it in 38 years. "I really did it to alleviate the stress," he said. "Darn, if it didn't feel pretty good!"

At the 2001 National Masters Track & Field Championships in Baton Rouge, Vaughn told me of his conversion from couch potato to one of the top over-60 shot putters in the country. He had thrown at the University

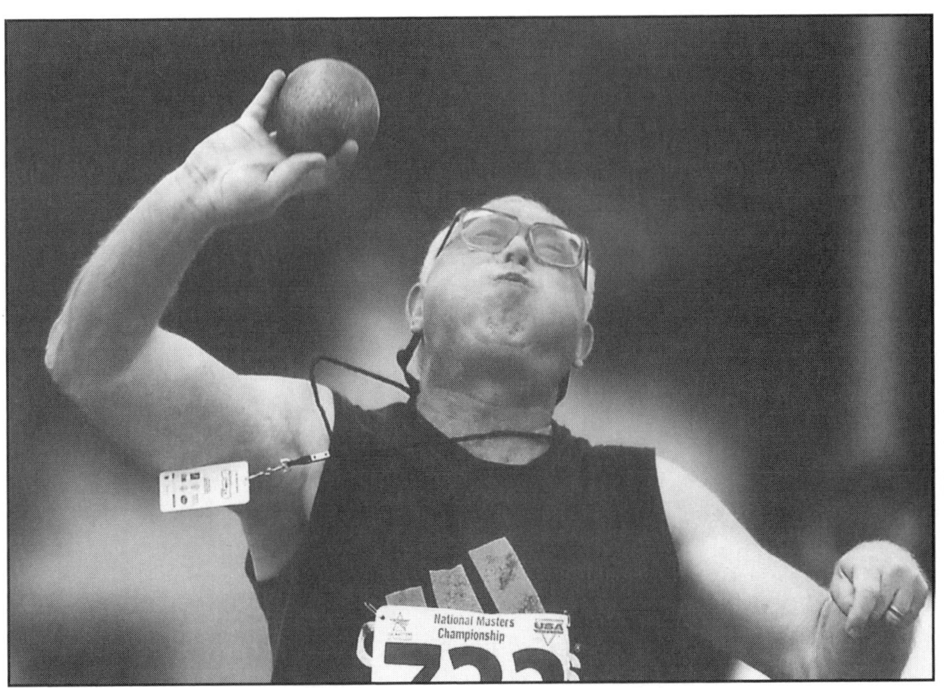

Photo courtesy of William E. Vaughn, Jr.

Gerald Vaughn's strategy for shot put: Each throw must be "violent."

of Richmond but had a middling collegiate career. A friend at Harvard was throwing 10 feet (about 3 m) farther at the same time.

When Vaughn started back again, he began throwing with Floyd "Chunk" Simmons, a fellow resident of Charlotte, North Carolina. Simmons was a bronze medalist in the decathlon in the 1948 and 1952 Olympics. "Chunk told me, 'Jerry, you're good,' and that's all he had to say," Vaughn recalled. "But he told me that I was going to have to lift weights."

By that time, Vaughn's wife had died. His children were married and he was coming home to an empty house. "I really needed to work out because I had nothing at home," he said. "That motivated me to really practice."

He started slowly, but he began lifting more and more weight. "I was doing phenomenal things in the weight room," he told me matter-of-factly. The year before we met, in 2000, he lifted 6.5 million pounds (almost 3 million kg) with his upper body and 8.1 million pounds (about 3.7 million kg) with his lower body. He threw the shot 4,005 times. His goal was 4,000 times a year, so a week before the end of a month, if he wasn't on

Internet Resources for Masters Athletes

Clarence Bass—Bodybuilding & Fitness Home Page: www.cbass.com

European Veterans Athletic Association (track and field): www.evaa.ch

Fédération Internationale de Natation [International Swimming Federation]: www.fina.org

International Masters' Speed Skating Committee / ISU Masters' Speed Skating Working Group: www.imssc.org

International Powerlifting Federation: www.powerlifting-ipf.com

Masters Athlete magazine: www.masters-athlete.com

Masters Athlete Physiology and Performance: http://home.hia.no/~stephens

Masters Athletics (track and field): www.mastersathletics.net

MastersTrack.com: www.masterstrack.com

National Masters News: www.nationalmastersnews.com

The President's Challenge—Adult Fitness Test: www.adultfitnesstest.org

United States Masters Swimming: www.usms.org

USA Powerlifting: www.usapowerlifting.com

USA Triathlon: www.usatriathlon.org

World Masters Athletics (track and field): www.world-masters-athletics.org

schedule, he would walk into his backyard where he had built a shot put ring and start throwing. "However many it takes to get to that total, I will do it," he told me.

At 65, Vaughn was 6-foot-3 (190.5 cm) and weighed 250 pounds (113 kg). His massive biceps were punctuated with Harley-Davidson tattoos on each arm. By outward appearances, he was a man you didn't want to mess with. But seated in the stands of a gymnasium at Louisiana State University, Vaughn was a Southern gentleman with a playful air. The tattoos, he told me with a wink, were pasted on to psyche out the competition. "I want them to think that I am rough and tough," he said.

Each year he trained harder. And each year he got better. He was convinced he would break records in the shot for years to come. "I have not had the perfect throw—not even once," he said. Once a thrower has developed good technique and strength and mastered the art of pushing a heavy ball as far as possible, "you should have a perfect throw one or two times a season," he said. "I haven't had a single perfect throw. That's what I am working toward."

Vaughn, a retired human resources manager, remarried two years after his wife died. His new wife, Becki, a runner who competes in 10Ks and marathons, also took up the shot and is nationally ranked in the 60-to-64 age group. They met through a family connection: Becki, whose husband died in 1990, is the mother of Vaughn's son-in-law.

In 2007 when I caught up with him, Vaughn was nearly 72 and weighed 265 pounds. He had added 15 pounds (6.8 kg) of muscle. In six years, he had become stronger and was throwing the shot farther.

Vaughn doesn't lift free weights and relies instead on weight machines to reduce the chance of injury. He also wears braces on his wrists. He doesn't try to muster up a single big lift. Rather, he lifts as much as he can as many times and as fast as he can because the shot requires power and quickness. "Everything is fast because I want those fast-twitch muscles," he said. He does about 20 different lifts at the gym. In the fall of 2007, for the vertical chest press, which is like a bench press, Vaughn was lifting 285 pounds (129 kg) 59 times. (The weight on a machine is lighter than free weights.)

When he was getting ready for a big meet, he moved from his maintenance stage to doing three sets of all of the lifts as many times as he could. Even though he was lifting more, Vaughn had cut back on his throwing to once a week. He tried to pick a day that had weather conditions similar to what he might be facing in actual competition. After he warmed up, all of his throws were at maximum intensity. "I say to myself that each such throw is going to be violent," he said.

Vaughn has been USA Track & Field age-group champion, indoor and outdoor, eight consecutive years, including 2008. He has broken the world outdoor record three years in a row and held three world indoor records. With time, he has learned that achieving perfection is harder than he thought. In 2007, he traveled 13,000 miles (21,000 km) to compete in 19 meets. He competed so much because, despite his training, "exceptional" performance can be achieved, he believed, only 10 to 15 percent of the time.

Then in Winston-Salem, North Carolina, in 2006, he tossed a 4-kilogram (8.8-pound) shot 52 feet, 4.5 inches (almost 16 m)—nearly two feet farther than he had ever thrown before. A USATF-certified official was on hand to measure the throw. It should have been a world record, but the meet had not been sanctioned by USA Track & Field. Vaughn finally got his perfect throw, however. The shot seemed to glide off his hand. It felt, he said, "like a feather."

3

Older and Faster

By the time they were 50, all three men were turning back the hands of time.

Jim McConica, the best of them in his younger years, was swimming better than at any time in a decade. Greg Shaw, who swam briefly in college before dropping out, was simply faster than at any other time in his life. The same was true for Trip Hedrick. His times were all the more impressive because Hedrick had come back after suffering a heart attack at 46.

All three swimmers were at the top of their game. Each had set world records in their 50s, and in their own ways they believed they could continue to improve. They are vivid examples of the possibility of maintaining peak athletic performance well into middle age. McConica, Shaw, and Hedrick are certainly outliers—their achievements go far beyond the reach of most of the rest of us. But what older athletes and researchers are finding is that diligent exercise can act as a biological brake on the aging process.

"Thirty years ago when masters swimming was just getting started, we didn't really have a clear concept of what we could achieve as we aged," said Bill Volckening, editor of *USMS Swimmer* magazine. "Now we are just hitting the tip of the iceberg."

UNDERESTIMATING THE AGING ATHLETE

Dara Torres personifies the undiminished powers of an over-40 athlete. In 2007, she won the national championship in the 50- and 100-meter freestyle and finished second in the 50-meter freestyle at the FINA World Cup in Berlin. Her time of 23.82 seconds in the World Championships was an American record—two seconds faster than her time in 1984 when she made her first Olympic team. At the 2008 Olympics in Beijing, swimming against women who were half her age, she won three silver medals: the 50-meter freestyle, 400-meter freestyle relay, and 400-meter medley relay.

"I think," said long-time swimming observer Phillip Whitten, "that we've underestimated people's abilities as we age." Whitten, former chief media officer of *Swimming World* magazine and currently executive director of the College Swimming Coaches Association of America, believes times of older swimmers could be even faster. The limiting factor isn't so much the failure to tap undiscovered training secrets—it's the reality of everyday life that is the limiting factor. Most adults can't afford to train more than two hours a day. They have to hold down jobs, take care of families, and stay mentally focused for so many years.

Torres, a neophyte in the aging game, has financial support from sponsors to bankroll $100,000 in annual training expenses, which include two swim coaches, a strength and conditioning coach, a pair of stretching coaches, a masseuse, a physical therapist, a diet consultant, and a nanny for her daughter. Neither Shaw nor Hedrick enjoys such luxuries, and neither man devotes the kind of pool time required of an Olympic hopeful. McConica gets closer. His workouts are legendary. In 2004, one session in the pool lasted more than eight hours. The same year, in February, he swam 300 miles (483 km)—an average of more than 10 miles a day—as part of an annual winter fitness challenge in which swimmers see who can log the most distance in the pool. He was edged out by Jewell Grigsby-Martin of Virginia, who swam 301 miles. Grigsby-Martin was 72.

"The biggest thing, I think, is the mental attitude," McConica said. "We don't have to be old yet—I don't want to cave into old age. My mental capacity is much better now than it was when I was younger. So is my threshold for pain to get through tougher workouts."

JIM McCONICA: I DON'T LIKE FAILURE

When I first met McConica (born in 1950) at a swim meet at the George F. Haines International Swim Center in Santa Clara, California, in 2001, he was 50, recently divorced, and the owner of an auto dealership in Ventura, California. He was trying his best to attend two-a-day practices with the Buenaventura Swim Club, a youth team.

"The coaches get a lot more out of me than when I was in college," he said. "We're doing different things all of the time. You get challenged at different times during a workout. I think that really helps."

At 52, McConica's times in three disparate events—the 200-meter freestyle, the 1,500-meter freestyle, and the 400-meter individual medley (butterfly, backstroke, breaststroke, and freestyle)—were all faster than when he was 42 when he was still one of the best in his age group. A look at his performances is instructive. McConica was no longer swimming as fast in a sprint event such as the 100-meter freestyle. But his time in the 200-meter freestyle was quicker. He swam 2:03.94 compared to 2:05.26 when he was 42. In the long-distance 1,500-meter freestyle, he swam 17:27.75—20 seconds faster than 10 years earlier. And in the multidisciplinary 400-meter IM, his 5:07.52 was nine seconds faster. The older McConica was training smarter and often swimming harder than he had been a decade earlier.

Since our first meeting, McConica has been able to spend even more time swimming. In 2004, he sold his auto dealership and devoted attention to various projects, including fund-raising for a new multimillion-dollar recreational park in Ventura. The next year, he applied to become an ocean lifeguard for Los Angeles County, won the swimming portion of the test, and started patrolling Southern California beaches.

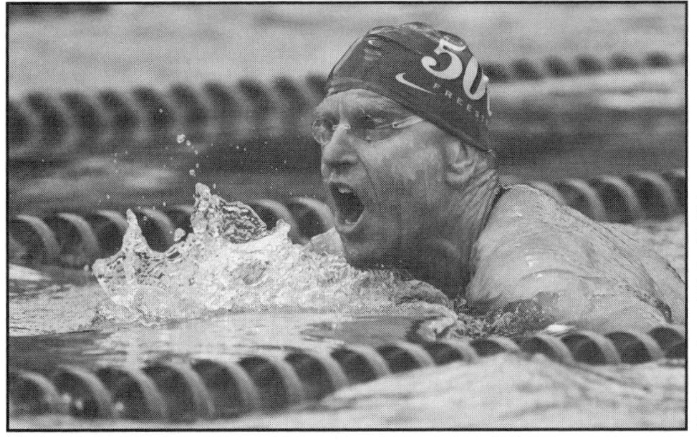

Photo courtesy of Peter H. Bick

Jim McConica believes training with a youth swim team has made him faster.

Swimming as the Fountain of Youth

Older and Faster

Phillip Whitten wanted to better understand the relationship between aging and physical activity. For years, he watched instances where the times of men and women barely changed as they got older. Some were even swimming faster.

Researchers had long held that most people peak in strength, speed, and oxygen uptake at the age of 25 and then drop 1 percent every year afterward. Whitten compared the times of the same swimmers from 1975 to 2000, using the 100-meter freestyle—an event unfettered by rule changes that tend to improve times. The 100 free is also the most popular event and requires the use of both aerobic and anaerobic energy.

Whitten found that men and women improve between the ages of 25 and 40 and don't begin to decline until after age 40. In their early 40s, swimmers begin to experience an imperceptible decline of .16 percent per year. Between ages 40 and 50, the annual decline is about .25 percent; between 50 and 60, the drop is about .66 percent a year. Preliminary results were first published in the July/August 1992 issue of *Swim* magazine and later updated in the March 2005 issue of *Swimming World* in an article titled "Holding Back the Years: How Much Should We Decline With Age?"

The 1 percent rule, Whitten concluded, applies only to people who are sedentary. "What it means is that if you live a typical sedentary American life, you will lose about 25 percent of your physical capacity by your 50th birthday. By your early 70s, you will be half the man or woman you were at 25. In contrast, if you swim regularly, the decline is only 3.9 percent at age 50 and 20.9 percent at 70."

Swimming and a Better life

Joel Stager, a professor of kinesiology and director of the Counsilman Center for the Science of Swimming at Indiana University, has observed the same thing and has come to conclusions similar to Whitten. In his studies of masters swimmers, Stager used biological measures: body mass, blood pressure, blood chemistry, handgrip, vertical jump, skinfold measurements, and pulmonary function.

Swimmers had a lower risk of cardiovascular disease with lower triglycerides, cholesterol, and blood pressure. They also scored better in the vertical jump (a measure of power), muscle mass, and pulmonary function. Stager, a competitive masters swimmer, asserts that active middle-aged people are in some ways closer to Americans of 100 years ago than their couch-bound contemporaries. "If we were all out there getting the cows out at 5:30 in the morning and closing up shop at 9:00 at night, maybe everybody would be like this," he said.

In Palo Alto, California, at the FINA Masters World Championships at Stanford in 2006, Stager's staff had just finished testing a male swimmer with a pulmonary function that was 36 percent above normal. The man, who looked to be in his 60s, asked whether it was a good score. Stager said it was very good. (Masters swimmers who were tested for pulmonary function by Stager averaged 15 percent above normal.) Then the swimmer asked if anyone had gotten a score that was 50 percent above normal.

"That's so typical," Stager said, smiling and shaking his head. "That's the psyche of this group. These guys want to know what's the best."

Most men and women can't quit their day jobs, but they are helped by swimming's highly developed organizational structure: The need for a pool brings people together. Many communities have masters swim clubs where workouts are overseen by a coach. Training techniques continue to get better. And much of the latest know-how is handed down from the elite to the masters ranks. Swimmers can also attend camps, rent or buy instructional tapes, or learn through books and magazines about how to train or tweak their strokes. Each year, a dozen top masters swimmers are invited to the U.S. Olympic Training Center in Colorado Springs to take on the persona of an Olympic athlete. In addition to classroom instruction, their strokes are dissected in a 50-meter pool and in an aquatic research flume—a treadmill for swimmers. As they swim, they are filmed with an underwater camera and periodically poked with a needle so that their blood can be tested for lactic acid, which helps researchers assess their level of conditioning.

Swimmers also benefit from sport-specific improvements: Suits are manufactured for less resistance in the water, and gutters and lane-line markers are designed to absorb wave action better and let swimmers move faster.

McConica has leveraged training and technology to get better. He began working out with high school swimmers in his late 40s. Even though he had been one of the best in his age group, "I was going backward," he told me in 2001. "I was up to right around five minutes for the 500 (freestyle) and that wasn't satisfactory for me. Today (three years later), I swim it in 4:47. The key has been training with these kids. It's a great environment for me. I'm able to compete head up with most of them. Somebody's got to touch the wall first, and I like to try to touch the wall first."

McConica joined the team while he was still running his dealership. He had to be in the pool on Mondays, Wednesdays, and Fridays by 5:00 a.m. and swim until 6:30 or 6:45. On Tuesdays and Wednesdays, he was there from 6:00 to 7:00 a.m. He also tried to join them for an hour of practice at night. On Saturdays, workouts lasted two hours in the morning. "There are trade-offs every day," he said. "The toughest part for me is making it to the pool. If I waver at all, that's my day."

Had he been married or had his children been living at home, it would have been much harder. And had he been training alone or with people his own age, "then you have to make yourself reach down—instead someone else is reaching down and pulling you along," he said. "I'm benefiting by competing every day." For a time he had been putting in as much as 50,000 yards (45,720 m) a week—28 miles, or 45 km—a staggering amount of work. In 2000, he dropped down to 30,000 to 35,000 yards (27,430 to 32,000 m), far more than most masters.

McConica was also doing open-water swims. In 2004, at 53, he made his third crossing from Catalina Island to the coast, a distance of 21 miles (34 km). He had broken the record in 1983 at age 32 in a time of 8:27:24 and held the record for a decade. McConica has also swum the English

A Masters Workout

Most masters swimmers who compete in meets will swim an average of 3,200 to 3,500 yards (about 2,930 to 3,200 m) a day and train three to five days a week (3,200 yards is 128 lengths of a 25-yard pool), Masters swimmers will typically dial up their distance and intensity once a week.

Bill Volckening, a former masters coach and editor of *USMS Swimmer* magazine, offers the following workout. Total distance is 4,200 yards (3,749 m).

Set category	Set description	Set intervals
Warm-up	100-yard freestyle, 100 kick, 100 pull, 50 drill (repeat).	No rest.
Kick set	12 × 50 yards in IM order: butterfly, backstroke, breaststroke, and freestyle.	Rest 20 seconds between repeats.
Preset	400 yards freestyle, starting slower and finishing fast. Don't worry about a fast turnover rate. Keep long arm stroke.	No rest.
Main set	10- × 200-yard freestyle, starting moderately fast and ending fast in the first 5. In the second 5, do the same, but try to end up swimming faster.	Allow 15 to 20 seconds rest on the first 200. Rest increases as speed increases.
Cool-down	8 × 50 yards, 25 drill/25 freestyle. Slow and easy.	Rest 15 to 20 seconds between repeats.

Pull means swimming without kicking. Pull is often done with a pull-buoy for leg flotation. *Drill* is any number of exercises that isolate a specific phase or movement of a stroke (for example, swimming with hands closed).

Channel. One of his goals is to become the oldest man to cross it. (The current record is 67.) His sole interest in trying to swim the Catalina Channel a third time was his belief that he could take back the record.

On an October night, McConica and his crew left shore a few minutes before midnight. The ocean temperature was in the mid-60s. The water was clear and he could see large fish swimming under him. At one point, he had eye contact with one fish that was as large as a shark. Jellyfish stung him again and again like a thousand paper cuts. But there were also playful dolphins and the light show of the phosphorescence of the fish below him. However, the ocean currents changed and threw him off course. His hope for swimming the channel in record time was fading. He fought seasickness, a searing headache, and hypothermia.

"When those negative thoughts started coming, I worked very hard to get my mind right," he wrote in a personal account in *Swimming World*. "I used every trick I know to get through those bad times. I thought of inspirational people who have persevered through tough times. I thought about focus and pride. Pain is temporary. I am not going to die—I just felt like it."

He finished in 10:19:24. Motivation can come from many sources, and McConica seems to find it wherever he can. He told me he is happiest when he is around water. At Santa Clara in 2001, I watched him walk through the stands like a town mayor. He made a special effort to enter an early race so he had time to wander around and meet old friends. He's lanky: 6-foot-3 and 185 pounds (190.5 cm and 84 kg). Every few feet, he would stop, shake hands, exchange pleasantries, and move on. He did the same in 2006 at the world meet at Stanford—an ocean lifeguard telling stories to his buddies about life on the beach.

McConica swam at the University of Southern California, where he developed mightily from an underperforming freshman to a national champion. He was NCAA champion in the 200-meter freestyle in 1971 and 1973. Mark Spitz was the first to swim under two minutes in the 200. McConica was the second. But at the 1972 Olympic Trials, in the 200, his best event, he missed making the team by .10 of a second.

"I was very close," he told me, "but close doesn't work. That is part of my motivation. I don't like failure. And that was failure for me." Had McConica made the U.S. squad, he would have been on a relay team that won a gold medal in Munich. "I should have been on the team in 1972, and I would have gotten a gold medal," he said.

Another source of inspiration is a friend and former training partner who died of cancer. So are the kids on his swim team. At Santa Clara, he seemed like a man on the verge of a heart attack after he staggered out of the pool, gasping for breath after swimming the 500-meter freestyle.

"I was in distress," he said. "If you are not hurting like that, you haven't gone all of the way down where you need to go."

Adapted, by permission, from J. McConica, 2004, "Jim McConica recounts his toughest swim: From Catalina to the U.S. mainland," *Swimming World*, Nov. 1, 2004. Article is available for purchase at www.swimmingworldmagazine.com.

GREG SHAW: FROM PLATO TO THE POOL

Greg Shaw, who shares a birthday with McConica but is one year younger (born in 1951), recalled his own Olympic moment. It was his freshman year in college. He had been a star back home in Nebraska and had earned a swimming scholarship to Arizona State University. But the practices seemed tedious. He was burning out. He was on the pool deck after a morning practice when his coach asked, "Don't you want to be in the Olympics, son?" Shaw thought for a moment, looked at him, and said no.

He would stay out of competitive swimming for 30 years. Shaw gravitated to meditation practices and the counterculture. He went to graduate school and earned a doctorate from the University of California at Santa Barbara. Today he is a professor of religious studies at Stonehill College in

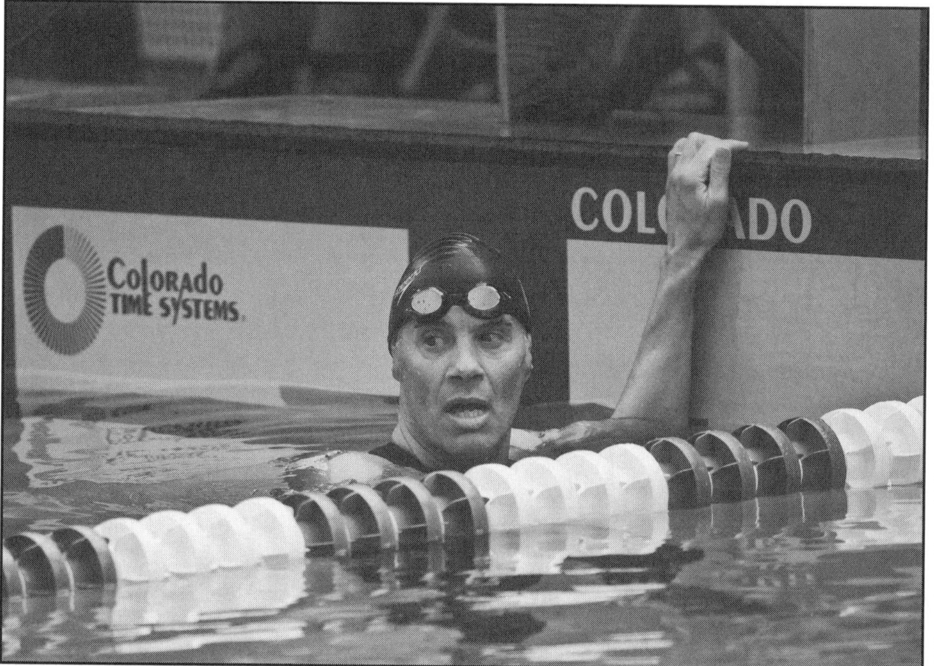

Photo courtesy of Peter H. Bick

Greg Shaw tries to create a mental image of swimming as much like a fish as possible.

Easton, Massachusetts, where he specializes in mysticism, neo-Platonism, and the origins of Western spirituality.

Shaw jogged and continued to swim, but not like in the old days. He'd knock off 16 lengths and head home. Then one day a fellow swimmer asked whether he would be interested in entering a masters competition. At 48, he entered a meet at Harvard. In his college days, swimmers hadn't started wearing goggles in races yet. At Harvard, he wasn't sure how to dive into the pool so that his goggles stayed on.

But he liked it. "I wanted to do something creative and distinct that I could really do well—outside of my day job," he said. "Maybe if I was into music, I would have gotten into a band. But it was this."

He was keeping track online of the top swimmers in his age group and was intrigued by McConica's ability to get better. Shaw began to entertain the same thoughts. Could he whittle down his times to those of his college days?

Shaw's wife, a runner, understood his return to the pool. His son and daughter, in their teens, were ambivalent, and his son thought it strange that middle-aged men would parade around in their Speedos. "They are more modest," Shaw said. "It's a different world." His colleagues, meanwhile, were polite, but their enthusiasm was tepid. "They're willing to hear about it once—but not twice," he said.

Swimming had changed from drudgery to a welcome release from the academic world. It was physically demanding but also deeply meditative. Other swimmers have told me similar things. They love the fluidity, the sense of weightlessness, or simply being away from the noise and bluster of life. "It's a sensory shift," Volckening said. "It's sensory stimulation. You are putting yourself into another type of atmosphere, really. There are definitely a lot of sensations you experience when you swim. You experience the feeling of the cool water, or if it's warm, warm. You experience the sound. You smell the chlorine in the pool or the salt in the ocean. You taste it. Actually I think that swimming involves more of the senses."

Shaw, the philosopher, was also drawn to the precision of it all. "In the academic world, it's not always entirely clear how well you are doing," he said. "In the pool, the measure is the clock. There is no ambiguity. It was a time when I needed some unambiguous feedback in my life." In 2003, at 51, he broke his first national record in the 50-yard butterfly. "I got hungry," he recalled. "Getting that record was like feeding a monster."

The next year in Indianapolis at the U.S. Masters Short Course National Championships, he swam the 100-yard butterfly in 53.6 seconds. He finished second, but it was his fastest time ever in the event. In high school, he had swum 53.8; at Arizona State, he had lowered it to 53.7

"I am much more conscious about how my stroke is working than when I was 18 or 19," he said. "I am much more aware of my rhythm. Back then I just did it."

Shaw swims alone in the afternoon for an hour a day, six days a week, at a YMCA in Bridgewater, Massachusetts, south of Boston. Afterward, he lifts weights for 15 or 20 minutes. He divides workouts in 1,000-meter increments, swimming, for example, 100 meters 10 times or 200 meters 5 times. When he gets closer to a meet, he tries negative splits—swimming the final sets at increasingly faster times. But he swims about only half the distance of McConica, an endurance specialist.

Shaw also traces each race in his head—each stroke, the turn, the breathing, he creates an image of moving through the water as fishlike as possible. "I think that the best competitive swimmers are able to get into a deep state of focus," he said. "And that requires a complete mental, physical, and emotional focus all at once. It's all consuming." He pushes aside all of the other distractions. He tries, he told me, to root out the "head case" raging inside of him.

There were no signs of anxiety at the masters meet at Stanford in 2006. He looked calm and focused before he dived into the water in the 100-meter freestyle. He finished second to a Norwegian, less than a quarter of a second off the world record, but ahead of former Olympian Gary Hall Sr., the father of Olympian Gary Hall Jr. When he pulled himself out of the water, exhausted, he listed across the deck, his arms swaying in front of him as if he were John Wayne in a swimsuit.

After his swim, we sat on the grass in the shade as men and women sauntered by in various states of undress. Shaw is lean and broad shouldered with gray hair, which turns silver at his temples. He didn't know how long he would keep competing. (Though a year later, despite a shoulder injury, he was named by *Swim* magazine as one of the 12 best masters swimmers in the world in 2007.) When he's had to deliver a major paper, he has struggled to keep everything in balance. He also wanted to write another book, his second. "If I have any good sense, I will keep competing until I'm a 100," he said. "There is no downside to this."

He told me in an e-mail a few days later that when he was competing in the 100-meter butterfly, "I may have had the best race of my life." The butterfly, graceful, undulating, and fast, is Shaw's favorite stroke. He has a knack for it. When things are working, he told me he feels as if he is gliding through the water. Many of his swimming friends know more about stroke mechanics and don't hesitate to point out his flaws. "But they usually don't tell me there's anything wrong with my fly," he said. "'Oh, your fly is fine—it works.'"

The race started "long, smooth, and fast," but he began to lose cadence and he started breathing on every stroke. He worried about the turn, but he timed it right. His pattern of breathing on every other stroke returned. Then in the final yards he found himself fading. He desperately wanted to lift his head from the water and breathe, but it would slow him down. "I was losing rhythm, energy, strength . . . just in time," he said.

He looked up and saw 1:01.05. He was 54 years old. He had never swum faster.

TRIP HEDRICK: FROM HEART ATTACK TO WORLD RECORD

In Indianapolis, when Greg Shaw swam the butterfly faster than he had in college or high school, the man who had beaten him was Trip Hedrick. Hedrick's time of 52.38 was also faster than he had swum in college. He was hot. He had swum 52.05 in Minnesota two weeks earlier, breaking the national record. All told, he had three other lifetime bests in 2004. Hedrick (born in 1954) was 50 years old and considered himself to be in the best shape of his life. It had been a remarkable year, and all the more so since he had suffered a heart attack four years earlier.

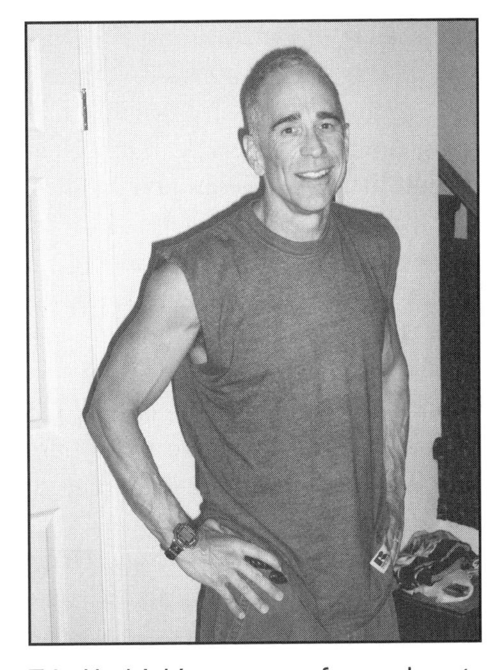

Trip Hedrick's recovery from a heart attack was both emotional and physical.

"I hadn't been feeling good," he told me in a spacious hotel suite he had booked for the meet at Stanford in 2006. Ever since the heart attack in 2000, Hedrick has paid closer attention to his diet. The suite helped. With a kitchen and two levels in which to move about, he and his wife, L'Louise, were able to cook for themselves and keep distractions to a minimum. "In hindsight, I hadn't been feeling right for six months," he said. "I thought it was battle fatigue from coaching."

Hedrick was the men's swim coach at Iowa State. His program had nearly been dropped twice for budgetary reasons. In 2001, the year after his heart attack, school officials eliminated the program.

One day while swimming, "I felt a little chest pressure and a radiating pain up my arm," he recalled. "It was enough to stop me and I thought this was a little weird. It went away. And a couple of days later, it happened again." He called his doctor and got a stress test. The results turned up nothing. But the doctor said there was a 20 percent chance the test could miss something. He continued to have what he called a "headache in my heart" and there were fleeting moments of chest pressure and acute pain.

Then on a brisk, cool day in May in the parking lot of a Target store in Ames, he was hit with a stiff gust of wind. For the first time he felt symptoms when he wasn't exercising. He went home, called his doctor, and went to the emergency room. Enzymes in a blood test showed no evidence of a heart attack, but the doctor recommended that Hedrick be taken by ambulance to Des Moines. Halfway there, he showed indications that he was having a heart attack and the ambulance sped down the road, quickly losing L'Louise in the car behind. The cardiologist at the hospital said he had 99 percent blockage of his left anterior descending artery. "You've had a heart attack and you have heart disease," he was told.

It was a shock. But he remembered how he once told one of his swimmers who had a benign brain tumor that doctors would take care of the medical problem. "It's the mental part of it that you will have to work on," Hedrick said. "I followed my own advice." (The swimmer went on to become an All-American.)

He started going to a counselor and he took a Myers-Briggs personality test. "I'm a feelings type of guy," he said. "It's very important for me to have everyone around me happy," which included 30 members of his swim team.

It wasn't entirely clear why Hedrick had blockage in his heart, but he was under a lot of stress and wasn't coping with it well. "Life stress, heart attack stress, event stress—the therapy was the best thing I did for my rehab," he said. "I had to learn not to sweat the small stuff as much."

Hedrick, sculpted by the pool and the weight room, was 5-foot-11 and weighed 165 pounds (180 cm, 75 kg) at Stanford. At the time of his heart attack, he weighed 190 pounds (86 kg). But he was strong, and he liked challenging his swimmers with pull-ups. He could pull his age until he was 43.

When he started his rehab, he suffered the indignity of being told to use only the weight of a broomstick on the bench press. He was accustomed to benching about 200 pounds. "This is going to be a problem," he told L'Louise. Beta-blockers, which control the body's response to high stress, were also prescribed, but they left him fatigued.

The Iowa State swim team went to Florida on a training trip during winter break and Hedrick learned that one of his buddies had entered him into a race among the coaches. He initially balked but decided to go ahead when someone lent him nitroglycerin, just in case. He swam surprisingly well. "That got me into the mind-set I could still compete," he said.

L'Louise, an elementary school teacher, is not a swimmer, but she enjoys going to the meets and making sure Trip is eating right and is well rested. "I was encouraging him to get back in the water," she said. "I knew it would be a good thing for him and I didn't think his demise was imminent."

Late Bloomer

Ironically, for someone who has stretched out his peak athleticism into his 50s, Hedrick didn't even swim in high school. As a freshman at the University of Kansas, he took an exhausting workout class involving running, weightlifting, and core-strengthening exercises—long before core work became popular. "Athletically, that's what made a man out of me," he said. In another course, he got his first structured swim training, taught by the Kansas swim coach. He picked up flip turns from his fraternity brothers who were on the swim team. By the end of the year, he wanted to keep swimming but wasn't so keen on Kansas. He transferred to Bemidji State University in northern Minnesota, joined the swim team, and became an NAIA All-American for three years.

He coached high school and was a graduate assistant coach at the University of Texas before moving to Iowa State. After the school ended its men's program, Hedrick went to work for Championship Productions, a company in Ames that produces and markets sport instructional videos. One of his responsibilities involves helping coaches distill their training secrets. He continues to coach Iowa State's summer swim camp.

After the heart attack, Hedrick changed his workout. His old routine included 2,000 to 3,000 yards of swimming on most days, followed by lifting weights. Now he exercises in smaller bites—30 to 40 minutes twice a day, or about 10 sessions a week. He swims five days a week, logging 1,500 to 2,000 yards. In addition, he lifts lighter weights one day on a circuit and heavier weights on another day. He has added Pilates, an interval workout on a treadmill, and running on stadium steps. The quick lifting, treadmill work, and stadium-step running are geared toward improving his cardiorespiratory system outside of the pool.

Intensity Counts

There is no magic formula for slowing down the aging clock. But the aging athletes I've met—the best ones—are always periodically pushing themselves as hard as they possibly can. For years Hedrick has done what he calls "keeping-me-honest" workouts in the pool and in the weight room. These workouts have specific targets, and his hitting them is proof positive that he isn't sliding backward. For example, in the weight room, he will move quickly through a dozen or so lifts, at prescribed weights, and perform 20 repetitions of each. After each round of lifts, he waits only a minute or two and goes at it again until he has completed three rounds and is exhausted. All told, it takes 35 or 40 minutes.

Although he may not receive the lavish attention Dara Torres enjoys, Hedrick's college connections provide him with the information that supplements his own considerable expertise. His swimming partner, Rick Sharp, is a professor of exercise physiology who was part of a team in 2007 that helped Speedo design a new high-tech swimsuit. His stroke coach, Duane Sorenson, is his friend and coach of the women's Iowa State swim team. One of his mentors is Eddie Reese, head swim coach at the University of Texas who coached the 2008 U.S. men's Olympic team, whom he talks with regularly.

Several factors drove Hedrick's comeback. His cardiologist told him it was all right to swim hard, which gave him confidence that his heart was strong. He's never doubted it since. Competition was a way of putting that confidence to a test. "I set some pretty lofty goals for myself," he said. "I wanted to see how far I had come back."

He'd always been a workout junkie, and in Hedrick's view, the prospect of easing off was stressful. "I don't behave very well, I get a little stir crazy, when I'm not working out," he said, looking at L'Louise. "Swimming has a very calming effect on me." And there was his coach's fascination with motivation. The heart attack represented the kind of challenge he was always telling his swimmers to confront and overcome. "I said this as a coach and I believe it now," he said. "Whatever sport you do, putting yourself in a position to fail—risking failure—makes you better. I think it's true for any part of your life."

At Stanford, Hedrick was stoic as he sat beneath a canopy on the deck and waited for his turn to swim. Then he and the other swimmers in his heat filed into the sunlight and snaked through the maw of dripping swimmers, photographers, officials, and onlookers. They climbed on to their blocks and fiddled with their goggles in the nervous moments before the start. Hedrick took first place in four events—the 50- and 100-meter freestyle and the 50- and 100-meter butterfly. With their smooth strokes and go-for-broke style, the best swimmers showed no signs of middle age. For these moments they were nothing more than swimmers. The best swam within a razor's edge of their best times ever.

This time, at the age of 52, Hedrick didn't swim his fastest ever. But in each race he came within hundredths of a second.

4

The American Birkebeiner

Barbara Klippel (born in 1933) often spends the early winter cross-country skiing on a flat trail near her home in Hayward, Wisconsin. It is nothing like the relentless hills on the American Birkebeiner course outside of town. Until the snow piles up, the big hills are too treacherous; they have to wait. Over the years, as much as she loved the Birkebeiner course, she'd had more than her share of troubles on it. A pine cone, upturned duff, an oak leaf—any of it—could send her toppling over. It had become harder to get up off the ground. Klippel would be 76 years old at the end of February 2009 when she planned to compete in her 20th Birkebeiner.

Among the more than 4,000 competitors who enter the 33.5-mile (54 km) race, Klippel would be the oldest female. Depending on the snow and her conditioning on race day, it would take six hours or more to wend her way through the forest before finishing in downtown Hayward.

Much like a marathon, the Birkie attracts all kinds of skiers. It courts the elite, since the race is on an international circuit. At the other end of the spectrum are people like Klippel, who are simply interested in finishing or are looking for ways to eke out improvement. For many, the attraction is the ritual of the training, getting together with friends, and spending a long day on the trail. "I do a lot of chattering on the course," she told me the first time we met. "I talk to everyone. My husband said that if I didn't talk so much, my times would be faster."

Klippel is also there to add another notch on her Birkie belt. Her goal is to join the Birchleggings Club, a group whose members have finished at least 20 races. The club is named in honor of Viking warriors in the 13th century who wore protective birch-covered leggings when they rescued the baby Prince Haakon from an invading force. The original race, which takes place in Norway, is the equivalent of the distance the warriors skied in order to carry the young prince, the future king of Norway, to safety.

Members of the club receive special purple bibs with gold piping. They wear them on race day as badges of fortitude. The long hours, unending hills, and cold can take their toll on anyone. Every year, skiers are carted off the course in snowmobiles, or done in by an injury or exhaustion.

Klippel should have knocked off her 20 Birkies by now. But one year her son got married close to the race, putting a crimp in her training. Another year she fractured her ankle while skiing. Another year she broke her arm on the trail. There was also a bout of pneumonia, and then cancer, and in June 2005, at a party, she stepped back to admire some artwork and fell backward down a flight of steps and fractured her skull.

By the time the next Birkie came around, Klippel was lucky to be on skis but in no shape to enter the race. In the summer of 2006, her husband, Jim, died unexpectedly. The following year, conditions were awful. While training a few days before the race, she encountered a sharp and icy descent on the trail. She was still recovering from the skull fracture, which had impaired her motor skills. The hill was too much. "I sat down on the top of the hill and cried," she said. "I just couldn't make myself go down that hill." She decided she would not enter the race that year.

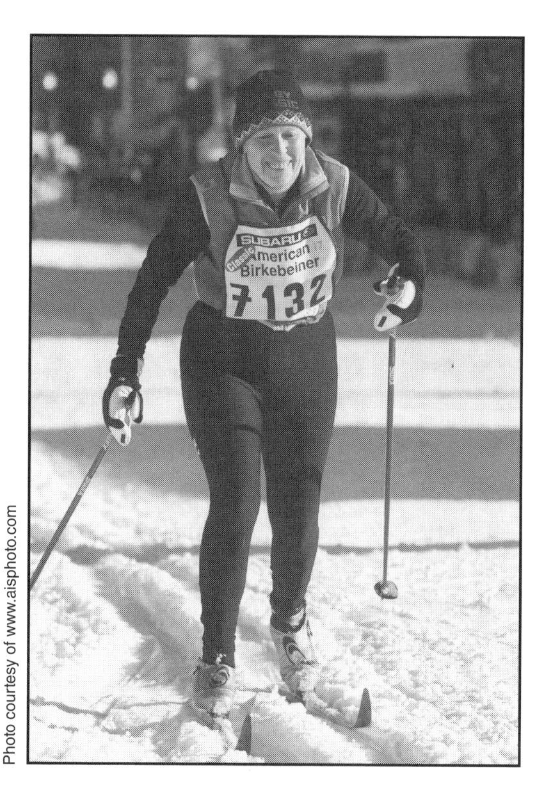

Photo courtesy of www.aisphoto.com

Barb Klippel approaches the finish line at the American Birkebeiner.

Another year passed. Her Christmas card in 2007 showed her decked out in her skiing garb and holding her poles and skis. The red-and-blue skis were plastered with decals from past

Birkie finishes. "Will I ever be able to wear the purple bib of a 20-year survivor of the marathon?" she asked. "I hope so." When I called her before Christmas, she told me, "It is *the* motivating factor for me right now."

"Barb is an extremely self-disciplined person," said her friend, Charlotte Duffy (born in 1933), who was then 74 and is six months younger than Klippel. "She is one of these persons who I swear is on the go all of the time. I couldn't live in her shoes for two weeks."

Ned Zuelsdorff, executive director of the American Birkebeiner Ski Foundation, believes many skiers use the Birkie as an inducement to stay in shape. He's found this especially so for older skiers. The average age of a Birkebeiner skier is 43, he said. About half the participants are between the ages of 40 and 59. "It is one of the things that keep older athletes going," he said. "You want to hold on to the fitness that you have and not lose anything so you can stay active—so you can be active."

When I met Russ Roberts at race headquarters in 2004, my second Birkie, he was getting ready to ski in his 27th. He was 65 years old and had moved to Hayward in 1996 so he could live near the course and train on it during the winter months.

"There isn't a lot you can do outside in the winter up here," he said. "There are snowmobiling and ice fishing. This is one thing that keeps me outdoors. Skiing the Birkebeiner, I think, really changes your overall lifestyle. I am not saying I'm in peak shape, but you make choices through the whole year that keep you in better condition. So when it's time to strap on the skis, you have a leg up." It was why he walked three miles round-trip to town every morning to buy a newspaper and why he always opted for the stairs over elevators. In the winter, he skied four days a week—6 to 20 miles a day to get ready. He's known Klippel for years, and if there wasn't enough snow locally, the two of them would drive several hours north to Michigan's Upper Peninsula.

A MARATHON OVER SNOW

The Birkie began in 1973 and drew 33 men and 1 woman. It was a time when skiers were flocking into parks and forests with their wineskins and wood skis. The era has had an unmistakable effect on the demographics of the sport. The style of dress and the technology have evolved. But there are still a few who cling to the roots of cross-country and glide along on wood skis in jeans and plaid mackinaws.

I entered my first Birkie when I was 48 years old and found it one of the hardest things I have ever done. The race begins on a barren field and, much as in a marathon, an elite corps of skiers bursts from the start.

With each successive wave, the skiers leave the relative warmth of heated tents, make a final check of the grip of their wax, and wait nervously for their start. A canon is shot and a great sea of bundled humanity surges forward across a canvas of snow. The rhythmic pounding of drummers pulls the skiers up the first hill before they disappear into the oblivion of the forest.

In the early going, the race is more like a morning commute—cold engines and overheated sports cars trying to get somewhere fast. On the first descent, a faster skier submarined me from behind and the two of us fell into a tangle of legs and skis and poles. My attacker said not a word and flew off, leaving me struggling to get back on my skis. I wasn't alone. There were wipeouts all around me and the mélange of styles and emotions made it difficult to settle into a rhythm. At the first few feeding stations, I rested and seethed while my ever-changing pod of skiers moved on. The feeding stops offered packets of energy gel, warm water and energy drinks, and partially frozen bananas and oranges. At one stop, I was treated to homemade chocolate-chip cookies. The goodwill helped assuage the jeers from beer-swigging snowmobilers who stood on a giant hill and delighted in watching wipeouts. I walked down the hill, which had been scraped by skiers in front of me to unnavigable hard pack. Depending on the weather, a Birkie skier has to contend with frostbite, hypothermia, sunburn, dehydration—or all of it. Snow conditions can change dramatically. After miles and miles of perfect glide, the bottoms of skis can turn to ice—or worse, sandpaper.

Despite the presence of thousands of skiers, the frenzy and zeal can be broken by moments of solitude. I would be alone for minutes at a time until another skier entered my universe. Slow folks like me with a late start time were rewarded with the rosy glow of twilight. It was a welcome sight—a light show that relieved a bit of the drudgery and a portent that the end was near. But sunsets and escape can also be easily ignored. It was still a race with hills to climb. The ever-changing relief is the defining character of the Birkebeiner. It is a remnant of the last great ice age, and all of the climbing takes its toll by day's end. "The hills, they just don't stop," Duffy reminded me in explaining why she no longer races. I paid a local ski shop $75 to wax my skis to make sure I was getting the optimal grip. If you've tried running up a wet, slippery slide, you have an idea of what the wrong wax does for you going up a hill. I was dog tired. I had skied maybe a half-dozen times before the race and depended on a six-mile run and few shorter runs each week in the preceding months to get ready. Head down, I had never looked at snow for so long and with such intensity.

The Birkie, Fat Tire, and a River Runs Through It

The American Birkebeiner (www.birkie.com) helped jump-start the Hayward area into a hotbed for aerobic-based sports. The race was the brainchild of Tony Wise, a local entrepreneur who owned a local ski hill. The ski hill is now closed, but the Birkie trail through northern forests offers the best cross-country skiing in the Midwest. In December 2008 *Master Athlete* named Hayward one the 10 best places in the United States for skiing. After the snow melts, the trail is used for walking, running, and mountain biking. Every September, cyclists pedal the Birkie in the Chequamegon Fat Tire Festival (www.cheqfattire.com)—the country's biggest off-road bicycle race. Other trails also thread the local forests for skiing, hiking, and mountain biking (www.cambatrails.org). In addition, the Namekagon River is part of a national scenic riverway and a mecca for canoeists and kayakers (www.nps.gov/sacn).

My spirit lifted in the final miles as I picked up the pace and started to reel people in. By the time I hit snow-covered Main Street with its cheering crowds, the Birkie had won me over and I could see why people keep coming back year after year.

THE LAST RACE

Each year the membership of the Birchleggings Club grows. On the eve of the 2009 race, there were nearly 850 members who had skied 20 or more Birkies. Elmer Hassett had desperately wanted to become a Birchlegger. He had been a career army man—a Nordic specialist who taught parachute jumping and cross-country skiing. During retirement, he built a cabin near the start of the course. "He was a tough old Norski," said an old friend, Dave Klostreich. "He loved the outdoor life. He was a true outdoorsman. He hiked. He snowshoed. He skied. His dream had been to find some land, build a cabin, and ski."

But in 1996 when Hassett set out for his 20th Birkie, he was suffering from prostate cancer that had spread to his bones. He made it to the halfway point, missed the cutoff time, and had to quit. The directors of the American Birkebeiner Ski Foundation offered him an honorary Birchleggings membership. But Hassett declined.

As the next year's race approached, he was no longer in condition to try again. But Hassett's minister, Lynn Larson, and another friend offered to carry him by sled. Once they got near the end, they would set him up on skis and let him finish the race.

"He pondered it for a while and then he shook his head and said no—he said it wouldn't work for him," said Larson, a Birchlegger himself. He is pastor of a Congregational United Church of Christ congregation in Cable, a small community near the start of the race. "Then he said, 'If I die before the Birkie, will you carry my ashes in your backpack?' I said I would be honored, if it came to that," Larson told me. Hassett died about a month before the race. He was 70 years old.

That year, 1997, Larson was 54 and skiing in his 13th Birkie. Hassett was a big man—6-foot-4 and 250 pounds (193 cm, 113 kg). The ashes weighed 10 pounds (almost 5 kg). To get used to the extra weight, Larson carried the ashes or loaded encyclopedias in his backpack on practice runs.

On race day, Larson wore his bib on his front and Hassett's bib on his back. Even with thousands of other skiers, the Birkie can be a long and lonely day. But this year, Larson had plenty of company. Three friends at the top of the first big hill yelled, "Push 'em, Elmer, push 'em!'" Along the course, skiers asked why he was wearing two bibs. Larson explained he was carrying the ashes of a friend who wanted to finish his 20th. "Some folks got teary-eyed, and of course, that affected me," he said.

And then there was Elmer himself. As Larson skied, he remembered how the old man used to complain about the weak church coffee, threatening to break away with his own branch of strong-coffee drinkers. It finally prompted Hassett to bring in his own Swedish blend. Then there was the time Hassett suggested that the church buy La-Z-Boy recliners so the service would be more comfortable. Larson reached the point in the race where in most years he was exhausted and ready to quit. He had skied for almost five hours. But now he didn't want it to end. He was not one, but two, skiers. "Sometimes I felt as if he were pushing me," Larson said. "I had never been a pallbearer before. For me, this was a spiritual journey to carry an old man's ashes."

Cross-country skiing is a sport divided by two different schools of technique. Klippel and I are traditionalists who employ the classic method of striding in tracks that line the perimeter of a groomed trail. The others, the faster-moving skaters, use a technique that commands the space of a country road. We are like Fords and Ferraris. At times, it feels as if the two groups represent an unholy alliance, codependent on their basic needs for space but disparaging of the other's approach.

THE EARLY YEARS

Klippel was in her late 40s when she began skiing with Charlotte Duffy and two other women. "After a while, there was a feeling that if you couldn't skate, you weren't successful," she said. "People were calling us the 'diagonaling dinosaurs,' but I didn't give a rip."

In one of the early years of the Birkie, Klippel watched skiers emerge from Lake Hayward and finish, and a few days later she told a friend, Sheila Wise, wife of American Birkebeiner founder Tony Wise, how much she enjoyed it. "Why weren't you skiing?" she asked Klippel. "I had visions of skiing the Birkie," Klippel told me, "but I didn't think I could."

Klippel had skied a little before then. She also played tennis, swam, and bicycled. But she had been reluctant to get serious about another sport until her son and two daughters were older. "In the early days, you are so involved in your kids' activities," she said. "You are an observer and not a participant." At their first Birkie, the women opted for the shorter 14-mile Kortelopet. The start was a forced march up a traditional ski hill; then they had to fly down the other side on their skinny skis.

Among her group, Klippel didn't shine in the beginning. But over time they all dropped out. Duffy, who still skis and bicycles, stopped doing the Birkie because it had become too difficult. "When we fall now and have to get up, it's a major ordeal because of the knees," she said. "My legs don't have the strength. Falling is a major thing."

Even for active women like Duffy and Klippel, balancing skills diminish over time. Arthritis (which robs joints of their flexibility), weaker muscles, and diminished eyesight are all common reasons. According to a 2008 report from the Centers for Disease Control and Prevention, falls are the leading cause of deaths and nonfatal injuries for people 65 and older. Each year, the agency says, one-third of older adults experience a fall.

To train before the snow flies, Klippel bicycles and hikes on the trail using hiking poles. She retired from teaching when she was 62; one reason was that it was getting harder to train. On Tuesdays, Wednesdays, and Thursdays she would ski a section of the trail—about 6 miles (10 km). On the weekends, she would ski 10 or so miles (16 km) in the early season and work up to 25 miles (40 km).

"Sometimes I would see the most beautiful sunsets," she said. "Sometimes I would end up skiing in the dark. I was skiing one night. I was cold. I was tired from teaching school. I thought, 'I could be out here during the day. I could retire now.' That's when I decided to retire." That fall, the first day of school, "I cried," she told me. "It was terrible. I went downtown and tried to relate to those white-haired people. And I thought, 'I'm not one of them.'"

Every year for the Birkie weekend, Klippel and her husband, Jim, would open their ranch home along the banks of the Namekagon River to family and old friends. Jim, a former downhill skier, worked at one of the feeding stations, and Barb cooked a pot of spaghetti for the prerace meal. In 2004, the first time I visited her, six inches of new snow had fallen and the thermometer hovered near the freezing mark. She had been working on her skis in the basement and worried about picking the right wax to match the changing conditions. She was thinking about driving to the New Moon ski shop a few miles away to hear what the wax company reps were recommending.

Klippel was the only woman in her 70s who skied the Birkie that year. She was 71. I wrote in my notebook, "Eyes twinkle." The next-oldest woman was 64. At 49, I would be skiing my second Birkie. I finished a mere six minutes ahead of Klippel.

"I have to be goal oriented; otherwise there would be no way I would be out there doing 30 kilometers of skiing when it's five degrees," Klippel said. "It's what keeps me going. As long as I keep beating someone, coming in ahead of someone who is younger than I am, I'll keep skiing."

At 51 she rode her bicycle across Iowa with one of her daughters. At 66 and 69, she hiked in and out of the Grand Canyon. For 13 summers, she helped lead a group that teaches English to high school students in Eastern Europe. After the Birkie, she would be on the phone and using e-mail to recruit teachers for the next trip.

We were sitting at her kitchen table when the phone rang. And then it rang again and again. Someone was looking for a room. Out-of-town callers wanted to know about the roads and the ski conditions. Guest Dean Rodeheaver walked into the kitchen from a downstairs bedroom. He was a gerontologist before becoming a college administrator. Rodeheaver told me that it was Barb's ego that was pushing her, and later he said, "This is really an identity issue with Barb. She really thinks of herself as a Birkie skier."

The late psychologist Erik Erikson described older adults like Klippel as those who looked at the accomplishments in their lives and were happy about them. Erikson was a personality theorist who believed that men and women begin to experience a sense of mortality at about the age of 60. This produces a period of introspection and reminiscence, and the outcome of this personal assessment can be positive or negative. In Klippel's case, it's been positive. "It's called ego integrity," Rodeheaver said. Those who can't reflect positively on their lives may find themselves struggling with despair and depression. They believe it's too late to change their lives.

Barb Klippel: In Her Own Words

On Training for the Birkie

"This is my job from the end of December through February. I think of it as a job—a very wonderful job."

On Taking Time Off After a Long Day of Skiing

"Instead of waiting one day for rest, I feel I should have two days of rest. It just takes longer to recover."

On Why She Is the Oldest Woman to Ski the Birkie

"It's just perseverance and strength of mind much more than it is strength of body."

On Her Recovery From Cancer

Each spring Klippel rides her bike to a patch of marsh marigolds along a stream that she noticed the first time after her diagnosis.

"It was a beautiful sight. If I hadn't had the treatment, I'd have never seen them. It's a marvelous feeling."

Ego integrity isn't necessarily built on a string of good fortune. In January 1985, Klippel felt that she was in the best shape of her adult life. In the previous summer she had competed in a local 50-mile bike race, the Firehouse 50. But then came her cancer diagnosis. It started with back problems. Then her head began to itch and burn. She thought she had picked up head lice from a student. Then her body broke out in a rash. One day she found a lump under her arm. A biopsy showed she had cancer.

"One night I got a call from my daughter telling me that we would be grandparents for the first time," she said. "A half-hour later, I got a call telling me that I had non-Hodgkin's lymphoma." She was 51.

Klippel taught kindergarten four days a week and drove to Duluth, Minnesota, on Fridays for chemotherapy. Her oncologist was optimistic. If she had not gotten treatment, she would have been dead in four months. With chemo, he estimated her chance of surviving at 40 to 60 percent. For months, she had no appetite and went through the day feeling as though she had morning sickness. But she eventually grew stronger and recovered. She had been treated with a man who was the same age and at the same stage of cancer and received the same treatment. He died.

In January 1998, she broke her right ankle skiing alone. "I started thinking about what I was going to make for dinner," she said. "You start wool gathering out there and you don't pay enough attention." Five miles from her car, she caught the tip of a ski in soft snow and fell. A physician passed by, examined her ankle, and concluded she would be fine if she iced it when she got home. She skied slowly back to the car and went to the emergency room; a doctor put her foot in a cast.

Another year, right before the Birkie, Klippel's ski hit a pine cone. The resin can act as a brake. She fell badly, broke her upper right arm, and tore ligaments in her shoulder. That year, she and Jim went to Arizona. "I couldn't stand being here for another Birkie, not being able to ski," she said.

Then, on June 5, 2005, at the high school graduation party of a former student, "I stepped backward to get a better look at some art—didn't even have a drink," she said. She fell down the steps into the basement and hit her head on the concrete floor. She remembers nothing, but later learned that she asked if she had fallen off her bike. She was taken by helicopter and then by ambulance to Duluth, where doctors removed a blood clot in her brain. She was in a coma for four days and spent five and a half weeks in the hospital.

"They said she wasn't going to make it," said Klippel's daughter, Sue Scheer. "And then they said in the best-case scenario, she would most likely be paralyzed on her right side."

When she came out of the coma, they asked her who the governor was. "I said, 'Minnesota or Wisconsin?'" Klippel recalled. "The doctor looked at my kids and said I was going to be OK."

"Mom had the advantage of being in really good health. That helped her endure the trauma," Scheer said. "I think it was perseverance and strength of mind as much or more than strength of body."

But it would be a long recovery. Klippel had also broken her collarbone and her left wrist in the fall. Doctors had to take a piece of bone out of her right hip to repair the wrist. She literally had to learn how to walk again. It wasn't until she returned home that she mastered getting off the floor by herself.

When I visited her for a second time in the winter of 2006, she complained about constant ringing in her ears. When she skied, she drooled out of the left side of her mouth. If she fell, she didn't have the strength and coordination to get off the ground without taking her skis off first. "I feel like a beached whale out there," she said.

She let me touch the right side of her head. The skin had grown back, but beneath the skin, it felt like a finger hole of a bowling ball. From there, I could trace a four-inch crescent where the doctors had removed part of skull to excise the blood clot.

A Pound of Prevention

Cross-country skiers, regardless of age, need to include strength and stretching exercises. Lee Borowski, former United States Ski and Snowboard Association Nordic Coach of the Year, is an author and cross-country ski coach. See his Web site at www.thesimplesecrets.com. He offers these tips for injury prevention:

- The strength element should cover the major lifts: Bench press and triceps press, chin-ups on a bar, lat machine or horizontal rows, military press for the shoulders, half squats or leg presses for the legs, and barbell or dumbbell curls for the biceps. Twice a week is best; the second session should be about 85 percent of the first session. Make sure you warm up first with a light set.
- Avoid being the overzealous trainer. A skier wants a lean build like a half-miler—not a shot putter. Despite the small amount of time I've spent on weights, I'm stronger now, at age 67, in every lift than when I was an athlete in college.
- Stretching should involve an assortment of exercises, including yoga and Pilates, that keep the muscles flexible, strengthen the core, and help you maintain your balance. A good one is the hamstring stretch. Lie on your back. Lift one leg and clasp your hand behind the knee and pull gently for about 10 breaths, then do the same with the next leg.
- You can do stretching for about 15 minutes one to three times a week. A good resource is *Back Rx* by Vijay Vad and Hilary Hinzmann.

Klippel seemed upbeat, given what she had endured. She wanted to keep skiing, but she hadn't deluded herself into thinking that she would pick up where she left off. "I know this is a slow process and I know that I have exceeded the expectations of the doctors," she said. "But I'm old. You don't bounce back as quickly."

That year, Dean Rodeheaver volunteered to ski with Klippel. She wore a bicycle helmet for protection. The two of them took part in a 7.5-mile (12 km) event, the equivalent of a fun run that organizers had started in the hope of attracting a new crop of skiers.

By the fall of 2007, she was getting ready for a full Birkie again. She walked the Birkie trail with her ski poles for practice. She had vacationed for two weeks in Mexico and walked and swum every day. Over the summer, she lived in Lithuania for a month to teach English—her 14th summer of teaching abroad. Afterward, she went to Poland for two weeks to visit former students. "This summer was a confidence builder for me," she said. "I could go ahead and teach and be away and do the things that I had done before my fall and do them successfully."

As fall gave way to winter, Charlotte Duffy joined her for skiing on the flat country in town. Duffy said it was still too early to say whether her old friend would knock off her 19th Birkie.

Klippel began training five days a week—an hour and a half at a time and longer on weekends. She never skied alone anymore. Daidre Bartz, who was 44, told Klippel that she would ski with her on race day. Bartz had begun skiing with Klippel and her own mother years before. Bartz's mom and Klippel had taught school together. "She knew everyone on the trail," Bartz recalled. "Everything gets pointed out to you. You'd stop and look at the trees. Everything was very much valued along the way. It wasn't so much that it was skiing as it was this adventure along the way."

Bartz's offer was a huge morale booster: "Just the thought that someone was going to be there who'd pick me up if I fell," Klippel told me.

Two weeks before the race, Klippel fell and injured her knee. A few days later, she and Bartz skied 11 miles. They had hoped to ski more, but Klippel was struggling. "It took us a very, very long time and when she got into the car, she had tears in her eyes," Bartz said. "She said she wasn't going to do the Birkie."

The injury would put her back another year. Eighteen Birkies. Two to go. Plus, Birkie organizers had made her the official starter of the 2008 race. A plaque she was given read, "You exemplify the spirit of the Birkie and you are a great ambassador for the sport of cross-country skiing." She'd have to stand at the starting tower, say a few words, and watch all of the jubilation around her.

She went to her doctor, who told her the race wouldn't cause further damage to her knee. Then another friend who had broken ribs skiing in Germany, and wasn't going to enter the Birkie, decided that he, too, would ski with Klippel. Another friend switched from the shorter Kortelopet to the Birkie to be with Klippel. A man from Green Bay joined in. So did a woman from Minneapolis. She had never entered the race but wanted to be with Klippel.

The local paper, the *Sawyer County Record*, called it Klippel's "flotilla." The group talked all the way and stopped at every feeding station to make sure she had enough to eat and drink. They scouted the hills ahead and decided the best route down. They walked two of the hills rather than risk a fall. One hill was the infamous junction of a snowmobile trail and the Birkie course, where the snowmobilers jeered skiers who fell or opted to walk down.

"We decided to all take our skis off," Bartz said. "They started booing us and we were all just thinking, 'Get us out of here.' And then one kid stepped out on to the trail. I think they had all been drinking and were having fun—not fun for us—but for them. He goes, 'Mrs. Klippel,' and gives her a big hug. Then they all start cheering us."

Klippel had been thinking about the final feeding station because Jim had always worked there. "That was sort of a milestone," she told me. From there, the course began to flatten out. The skiers crossed Lake Hayward. All that was left was the final few blocks on Main Street. One of Klippel's daughters ran alongside. The rest of her family was waiting at the finish. Her time of 7 hours and 48 minutes was almost two hours longer than the last time she finished the Birkie in 2005.

The next year, 2009, would not get off to a very good start. By early winter, Klippel was struggling with a foot injury. She had to undergo surgery to repair nerve damage and was forced to sit out the race. Although disappointed, she tells me that she isn't through yet. Her rehab is going well and in the coming spring she plans to enter a road race in South Carolina with her sister. Nineteen Birkies down, she still has one more to finish.

Part II

Defying Age

We all grow old. But some people age faster than others, and it's not just because of genetics. Exercise can reduce the inevitable deterioration that we'll all experience because it keeps our muscles and bones strong and improves our aerobic capacity. It even sharpens our balance. In some cases, good motivation and proper training means we can get better with age. The older athlete today has many advantages—improved healthcare, the democratization of training and sports medicine, and the power of numbers: Baby boomers are aging en masse, so there is a huge community of like-minded people to tap into. While it's true that America is growing more sedentary, older athletes have never had it better.

5

Fabulous Abs

For decades, Clarence Bass (born in 1937) has been photographed in bodybuilding poses that trace his transformation from an embryonic weightlifter of 15 to a ripped septuagenarian. The pictures represent a biological time line of how little the human body declines with proper care and feeding. His latest photographs, taken a few months shy of his 70th birthday, reveal a man virtually bereft of body fat. He is not so much a portrait of strength, though he is that; he is a model of muscle definition. Everything seems to pop. Tendons and veins rise up out of his skin like tightly drawn cables. He has abs to die for.

"For all of the softies of the world," said photographer Laszlo Bencze, who photographed Bass, "the only thing they desire is defined abs. And Clarence has got that in spades."

Outside the hypercritical eye of the bodybuilding establishment, where no imperfection goes unnoticed, Bass's physique has changed little since 1978 when he won his height class in the Past-40 Mr. America competition. The similarity between age 40 and 70 is all the more remarkable because Bass then was using anabolic steroids.

Now instead of drugs, he uses a few over-the-counter nutritional supplements. He lifts weights twice a week, mixes in another two days of short bouts of heart-pounding aerobics, takes lots of walks, and eats a near-vegetarian diet. He is not a slave to the gym. And when I spent a day with him in December 2007, we ate all day long.

America's health clubs are filled with barbell-lifting baby boomers intent on staying young forever. But will they, over decades, have the discipline, diet, and passion for weight training that Bass has demonstrated? Will any of them ever look as lean and strong?

"I don't think that you will ever see many people like Clarence Bass," said Terry Todd, a professor of exercise history at the University of Texas. "Clarence is very unique."

I learned about Bass when I came across his photographs in *Physical Dimensions of Aging* (1995), by Waneen W. Spirduso, a professor of kinesiology and public health, also at the University of Texas. Spirduso used pictures of Bass to make a point: Strength and muscular endurance decline mostly because of a lack of exercise—not because of factors associated with getting old. "One of the clearest findings in the literature on strength and aging is that disuse accelerates aging," she wrote.

For many years, much of the medical community failed to see the benefits of resistance training. "You really had to be there to see how people felt," said Todd, a former national champion powerlifter who weighed more than 300 pounds. He remembers meeting Kenneth Cooper, the physician and author of the 1968 book *Aerobics*. At the time, Cooper saw little benefit in strenuous weight training. But with new research, attitudes began to change. A 1998 study by the American College of Sports Medicine analyzed 250 research projects; among the findings, it found that strength training can make men and women stronger as they grow older, improve bone health, and help control weight. In one of the studies, older men and women were found to achieve greater gains in strength than younger people. Spirduso described elite elderly athletes as having a psyche in which the "body and its functioning are very important components of self-awareness and self-esteem."

When I first saw the photographs of Bass, I was impressed with how strong he looked. But his muscularity, at his age, seemed excessive. I

Aging Has Brought New Converts

In his newest book, *Great Expectations,* Clarence Bass offers his observations of health and fitness, leavened from the perspective of an athlete turned 70. As he's grown older and maintained his muscularity, he's found new converts. "I believe that's why many people relate to me now who didn't relate to me when I first appeared in *Muscle & Fitness* in the early '80s," he wrote. "I was younger and lean, but not young enough to appeal to guys in their 20s. But now that I am older—and still lean—and they're in their 40s, it's another story entirely. They identify with me now—and relate to my message. They can see themselves benefiting from my methods and example and, perhaps, in their own way, following in my footsteps."

thought about TV muscleman Jack LaLanne and the infomercials featuring impossibly strong men and women hawking the latest exercise device. Mind you, this was early in my research, and I hadn't yet studied anyone as muscular as Bass. I didn't fully understand the passion, pride, and ambition that drove the older athlete; I hadn't come around to the notion that if a 70-year-old man can sprint 100 meters or run a marathon, why couldn't he try seeking physical perfection?

"I think the primary reason people are uncomfortable about these sorts of muscle poses, and to some degree this is true, is that vanity and ego are on such public display," Todd told me. He is codirector of the University of Texas's Todd-McLean Physical Culture Collection, the largest archive in the world devoted to fitness, weightlifting, and exercise.

Todd described Bass as "sort of a poster child" for the older superfit and he planned on using photos depicting "the changelessness of Clarence's body" when the collection became the centerpiece of the university's new 27,000-square-foot Lutcher Stark Center for Physical Culture and Sports.

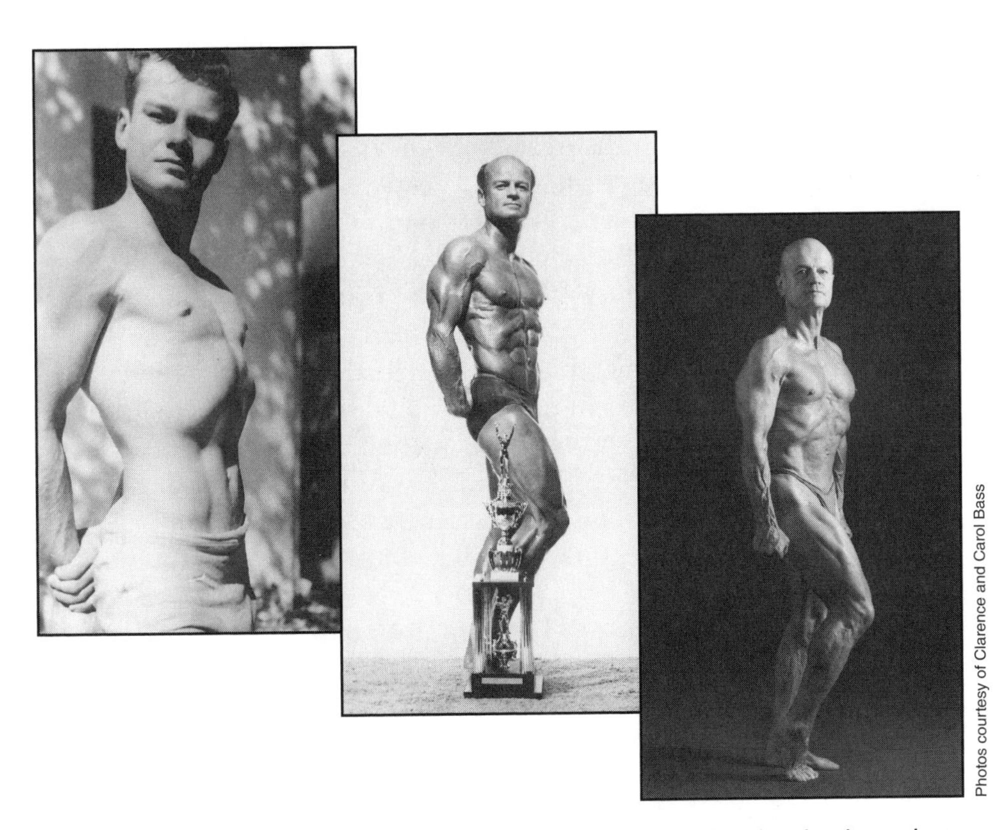

Clarence Bass at ages 15, 40, and 70. These photographs clearly show that his muscularity has changed little over time.

Muscularity can be intimidating, even when it's someone who qualifies for Social Security. "It's sort of like, 'What have you spent the last 30 years of your life doing? Well, not much,'" Bencze said. "And so that makes them feel guilty. And if you feel guilty, you are going to be angry."

HIS BODY OF WORK

In street clothes, Bass is lean and wiry. He is not tall—5-feet-6 (about 168 cm). His skin is remarkably smooth, and in certain light he appears 20 years younger. Bass is fond of sharing his views and, in fact, much of his time is now spent communicating his ideas on fitness. But it is with restraint—and not gimmicks. "He talks very softly but very strongly," said his old friend, Carl Miller, a former U.S. Olympic weightlifting coach.

"How I look is very important to me," Bass said when we first met at his home in Albuquerque, New Mexico. "That's my proof, so to speak." Photographs are the "most visible way I can show that I have maintained this level of fitness," he said. "I realize that it is a turnoff for some people who are not into bodybuilding. But one of the things that distinguishes me from almost any other bodybuilder is this continuing documentation."

Muscle definition is influenced chiefly by muscle size and level of body fat. Every Saturday morning before breakfast, Bass goes into the bathroom and steps on a scale that measures his weight and body fat. He records the changes in his neat handwriting on a legal pad, the numbers fluctuating by a pound and a tenth of a percentage point, respectively. He has tested his body this way since 1977. In the days before high-tech scales, Bass was dunked underwater in a laboratory by researchers at the Lovelace Foundation for Medical Education and Research in Albuquerque.

In his most recent photographs, Bass weighed 150 pounds (68 kg). His body fat registered 3.5 percent on his at-home scale—lower than that of most elite marathon runners. A more qualitative analysis occurs every morning when he gets out of bed and looks in the mirror at his nude body. "In terms of overall muscle mass, there are some poses that I used to be able to do that I can't now," he said. "But I am pretty proud of how I look."

Bass began lifting weights at 13, turning an old shed at home into his personal gym. As a junior in high school, he was New Mexico's state pentathlon champion—an event that combined push-ups, chin-ups, vertical jump, a 300-yard shuttle run, and an event called the bar vault, in which competitors pulled themselves over a high bar. As a senior, he finished second in the state wrestling tournament. In college, he began competing in Olympic-style lifts, which require quickness and strength. Then he took up bodybuilding.

The year after he won his height class in the Past-40 Mr. America, Bass, at 41, took first place in his class in another competition—the Past-40 Mr. USA. Overall, he won best abdominals, best legs, and most muscular man. He was in the best condition of his life.

Then he stopped competing and I wondered why he suddenly quit. "I might lose," he told me as we sat in his kitchen. "I really had nothing to gain and everything to lose. I developed my reputation with these photos, and these contests aren't a lot of fun."

Bass was practicing law full time. He was also writing a column for *Muscle & Fitness* magazine. The next goal was to leverage his credentials and write more expansively about weight training and bodybuilding. A year after leaving the posing stage, Bass wrote his first book, *Ripped: The Sensible Way to Achieve Ultimate Muscularity*, which he self-published in 1980. The book delved not only into his diet and training philosophies but also discussed his use of steroids. *Ripped* has sold about 55,000 copies.

Bass told readers how he had tried steroids without success during the 1960s to improve his Olympic-style lifts. "Frankly, I was skeptical, but as determined as I was to gain fat-free weight, I decided to give steroids another try," he said. For the Past-40 Mr. America, he got them with a prescription from his father, a physician who monitored his son's vitals. The steroids worked. They helped build muscle mass, and through a combination of diet and weight training, he whittled down his body fat to virtually nothing.

Bass's experimentation with steroids must be viewed in the context of the times. The International Olympic Committee added steroids to its list of banned substances for the 1976 Olympics in Montreal, but there was no testing for the presence of the drugs at bodybuilding competitions. It was certainly off the radar screen of professional sports and the public mind-set. In *Ripped*, Bass laid it out in the open. While he did not condemn those who used steroids, he concluded that even though he used them for a short time, they were a disaster on his body.

There are no known long-term effects of steroids because no studies have been done, according to Charles Yesalis, professor emeritus of health policy and administration at Pennsylvania State University and a leading expert on drug use in sports. "There has always been a vanity to man, but it is clearly accelerating," Yesalis said. "I think that performance-enhancing drugs are just one piece of the puzzle." Athletes use them to gain an edge, but there is also the human desire to look better. The use of makeup, tanning beds, cosmetic surgery, even exercise, all figure into this yearning for improvement, he said.

In 1978 for the Past-40 Mr. America, Bass had subsisted on a low-carbohydrate diet; in the weeks before the competition, he was eating 18 eggs a day. His hands trembled from overtraining. The diet, his training, and probably the steroids produced emotional highs and lows that he called his Dr. Jekyll and Mr. Hyde personality. With steroids, "in short, your body's hormone-producing mechanism gets lazy," he wrote. "Thus a real problem arises when you stop taking steroids."

As Bass was getting ready for his second over-40 competition without the aid of steroids, his body fat had zoomed from 2.4 to 9.1 percent. While still far leaner than the average man his age, he had six months to rid his body of unwanted fat.

Bass changed his exercise routine from megalifting sessions to shorter, high-intensity workouts that trained different muscles on different days. Each muscle group got four days of rest. He also reverted to a diet that leaned heavily on low-fat protein, whole grains, fruits, and vegetables. Without using steroids, he was able to increase his strength and reduce body fat. Bass has essentially stayed with the same whole-foods diet and workout regimen ever since.

"If you are going to be a lifetime trainer," he told me, "steroids are absolutely the wrong thing to do. You're just jerking yourself around." Bass also is not a proponent of two other potential aids for older athletes: supplements for alleviating declining testosterone levels or hormone-replacement therapy. He believes a good diet and exercise trump supplements' purported benefits without risking potential consequences.

Bass practiced law until he was 57. But as his interest in health grew, he went into the fitness business full time with his wife, Carol. He has written and self-published nine books; his latest is *Great Expectations: Health, Fitness, Leanness Without Suffering*, which was released in 2007. The couple has also produced five audiotapes and three DVDs. Their business, Ripped Enterprises, sells other products, including nutritional supplements. But unlike many fitness gurus, Bass does not tout supplements as the cornerstone of good health.

"The only defect with Clarence is that what he recommends isn't exotic enough," said Bencze, who in six months lost 20 pounds using Bass's whole-foods approach. With a good diet and exercise, Bass believes a person who wants to lose weight should try dropping no more than a half-pound (0.2 kg) per week. "It's so normal, so unweird that many people think it can't work," Bencze said.

EATING TO STAY LEAN

Bass rarely leaves Albuquerque and prefers to spend much of his time at his two-story stucco home where he answers letters and e-mails from customers and writes on the topics of health, diet, and exercise for his Web site, www.cbass.com.

I had been driven from my hotel to the couple's home by Carol, who was then 64 and whom he calls "the enabler." Warm and outgoing, she works from home in the morning and heads to the office in the afternoon mailing out products and handling administrative matters. She went back to college in her 60s, changed her major from biology to English, and edits her husband's writing. The couple has a son, Matt, in his mid-30s.

"I'm a control freak," Bass told me as he made me breakfast. "I don't like my routine to be broken. I don't want to have my training interfered with. In a way I have really an idyllic life."

Said Todd, "He would have probably made an ideal monk in the Middle Ages, up in a monastery in the hills of Greece, if he could have sneaked Carol in through the back door."

Staying close to home also allows Bass to control the food he eats. He is not a calorie counter, per se, but he has followed the subject so long that he knows the caloric value of nearly everything that goes into his mouth. He avoids food that contains concentrated calories, such as sugar and butter. He rarely eats red meat but also believes that a good diet is one that never calls for going hungry and allows for an occasional indulgence.

For breakfast, he scooped one cup of a mix of cooked oat groats, hulled barley, rye, spelt, kamut, and amaranth into a bowl and added two tablespoons of ground flax and a handful of frozen fruit. Then he poured in another handful of frozen corn, peas, and green beans and a cup of plain soy milk. Bass drinks both nonfat cow's milk and soy milk. But he likes soy milk because it has the fattier "mouth feel" of whole milk with fewer calories. He also prefers to use the sweetener Splenda, or sucralose, which cuts calories by reformulating the properties of cane sugar. He cooked the contents in the microwave.

He placed a huge bowl of food in front of me that looked absolutely awful. I love vegetables, but not in my cereal, and I am not sure I had ever tasted soy milk. On the table in front of me was a teaspoon. I was to eat this prodigious concoction not with a tablespoon but with a teaspoon. The idea was to slow down my consumption so I didn't eat past the point of feeling full. There was, however, an implicit understanding that I should finish the whole bowl. The breakfast turned out to be surprisingly good—nutty, sweet, and almost buttery. The grains gave it some heft and the fruit and vegetables went well together.

Later in the morning he offered me an apple. Bass often has an apple and a quarter-cup of salmon as a midmorning snack to keep his blood sugar at an even keel.

Fabulous Abs: Tips From Clarence Bass

Bass has a few key pointers on eating well to keep lean. It's all about control:

On Eating

Put on the table only what you are going to eat. This helps control the inclination to eat everything in sight.

Diets based on denial are psychologically flawed. If you tell yourself you can't have things, then you get those cravings and obsess over them.

Eating slightly less than what you burn is all that's necessary. The key is to eat foods that make you full and satisfied without taking in too many calories.

On Training

You should do some kind of exercise six days a week. Lift weights two of those days.

Walking is exercise. When combined with resistance training and more demanding aerobic routines, such as running or bicycling, walking becomes a form of active rest. It helps you recover from harder workouts.

To get stronger, you have to push yourself. Overload and rest. Boiled down to its essence, that is what training is all about.

On Aging

Active muscles have a faster metabolism than inactive muscles, regardless of age. If you stay active, you burn more calories.

It's a mind-set. I am trying to move forward. I may not be making progress on a grand scale. My muscle mass is not as good at 70 as it was at 40. But I do make improvements from workout to workout. That is my goal.

I have no plans on slowing down. I plan to keep doing this as long as I can.

Note: The above is based on Bass's conversations with the author and adapted from Great Expectations: Health, Fitness, Leanness Without Suffering, *by Clarence Bass, 2007.*

Before lunch we walked on a patchwork of trails on the eastern edge of Albuquerque that threaded through public land a few blocks from his home. Sometimes he and Carol will walk farther into the Sandia Mountains. Bass has timed himself getting to the top. He told me that he knocked 10 minutes off the climb when he began taking the supplement creatine, which supplies energy to muscles. He also takes a multivitamin and vitamins C and E. But this was a recovery day, and we walked leisurely through a moonscape flecked with withering grasses and cacti. On our return, the trail provided a sweeping vista of the city and the Rio Grande Valley.

"Most people think that aerobic exercise is boring," he said. "Well, the way most people do it, it is boring—going to gyms and reading newspapers. If you do it right, if you have a nice place to walk, you get revitalized."

When we came back, Bass served lunch: special peanut butter formulated with eggs and flaxseed and flaxseed oil on toasted whole-grain bread, a handful of carrots, and a large mug filled with equal portions of plain low-fat yogurt and plain soy milk. I was again handed a teaspoon. Bass quartered the sandwich for the same reason. "These are kind of mechanical ways to slow you down," he said.

By midafternoon, we were driving to his office in his Mercedes E55, and as I was eating a Tiger's Milk nutrition bar he had handed me, he gently admonished, "Eat slow."

Clarence and Carol often eat large salads, bread, and fish, chicken, or eggs for dinner. But that night we went to a restaurant that served traditional New Mexican cuisine. Carol, who is as lean as Clarence, ordered a large burrito, without cheese, and ate it all. Bass slowly polished off a plate of huevos rancheros, sunny-side up, and he shared a plate of Navajo fry bread with us. The two of them shared Mexican flan (custard that is drizzled with caramel sauce). Bass did not have any alcohol, although he occasionally will have a glass of wine. He is abstemious because "alcohol weakens the control I usually have over my appetite," he wrote in one of his books, *The Lean Advantage*. "It seems to anesthetize my stomach and encourage me to go on eating beyond the point where I would normally be full and satisfied."

For a snack at night, Bass has a slice of toast with almond butter, honey, and Benecol, a product intended to lower dietary cholesterol. He quarters the toast and eats a section every 15 minutes.

Bass felt he needed to drop 4 or 5 pounds (about 2 kg) and knock down his body fat by a few percentage points before he posed for his photos at 70. Six months before the shoot, he had preliminary photos taken. "I didn't like them," he said. "I had some extra weight around my love handles and lower back—pretty much everybody has it." He cut down by backing off slightly at every meal: a little less cooked grain and flaxseed at breakfast, smaller amounts of peanut butter, and one fewer slice of bread at dinner.

Ripped Enterprises is located in a one-story office building that housed his legal practice before Bass went into the health business full time. Two of the rooms are jammed with an array of weight machines, free weights, and other equipment positioned atop aging gold carpeting. The walls are covered with mirrors and posters of bodybuilders. One room is devoted to lower-body exercises; the other is for the upper body. There are plates, benches, cables, dumbbells, barbells, and a pair of weightlifting shoes. Each room contains impeccably maintained metallic blue Nautilus equipment from the 1970s that Bass bought from Arthur Jones, the founder of the company. Bass was so jazzed by the technology of pulleys and cams when it first came out that he and Carol flew to Florida to meet Jones.

He keeps additional equipment at home: In a room next to the garage, he has a Concept2 rowing machine, a stair stepper, a Schwinn Airdyne, and a Lifecycle. In his garage an entire bay is outfitted with a squat rack, old-fashioned kettle bells, weight-resistance machines powered by an air compressor, and a contraption called a glute-ham developer.

Bass had a heavy weight-training session the day before, his biggest of the week, so I didn't expect a big demonstration when we arrived at his

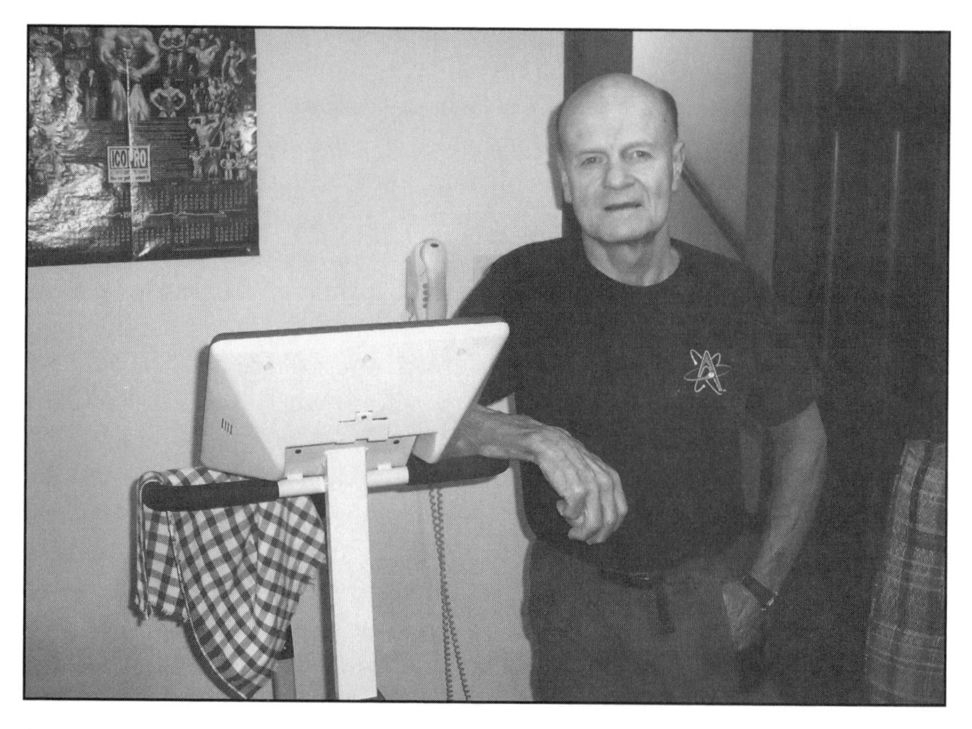

Clarence Bass at home where he spends most of his time researching and writing.

office. But when I asked about his favorite lifts to keep his abs so buff, he knelt down in front of a machine with a cable and pulley. He pulled down on the weight and let his oblique muscles do the work. At the bottom of the pull, he slowly raised the weight—again relying on his abdominal muscles. The exercise is often practiced with the subtlety of a pile driver. With Bass, it was almost sensual—an embrace between man and machine

"Clarence can't wait for the next workout," said Carl Miller, who owns a gym in Santa Fe. The key to lifting weights over many years "is that it has to capture your imagination so that you keep looking for ways to get better," Miller said. "You are always looking for a new training technique."

Bass has picked up and discarded an array of exercises and lifts over the years. At 60, for example, after more than a 30-year absence, he began incorporating technically difficult lifts such as the power clean and power snatch and squat snatch, which require quickness, strength, and good balance.

Bass exercises six or seven days a week, but he lifts weights only two of those days. He sits down with his workout diary before each session and plans what he will do. His diaries are 500 pages apiece and he's accumulated dozens of them over the years. Over time he has added more aerobic training for his cardiorespiratory system, as well. On periodic visits to the Cooper Aerobics Center in Dallas, his fitness as judged by tests on a treadmill or stationary bicycle consistently put him in the top category for his age.

Bass is a disciple of the HIT (high-intensity training) school of weight training. Early proponents included Jones (the Nautilus founder) and former world-champion bodybuilder Mike Mentzer. Advocates of HIT believe the best way to build muscle mass is with short, infrequent, but very hard workout sessions rather than hours of exercise almost every day.

Typically on Sundays, he will work his entire body with weights, making more than a dozen different lifts that push him to the upper end of his capabilities. After warming up, he will do only one heavy set for each lift—8 to 15 repetitions. "The key point is that I do not wear myself out before I get to the set that really counts," he told me.

Three days later, he lifts weights with his upper body then climbs on a Lifecycle, a computerized stationary bike, for 20 minutes and pedals hard at various resistance levels. By constantly changing the intervals and intensity, he is mimicking what he believes is humans' ancient need to exert short bursts of energy.

Three days later he does crunches and works sundry core muscles. He also does about 20 minutes of hard pedaling on his Aerodyne, which requires pedaling and back-and-forth arm action. On other days he goes on walks for 30 or 40 minutes.

Bass has pushed back the hands of the aging clock because of his triad of diet, aerobic exercise, and weightlifting. His metabolism burns calories as if he were a youngster because he continues to stay almost as active as one. Strong, exercised muscles, even when they are resting, burn more calories than less-trained muscles. "Anyone wanting to lose or control weight should, in addition to eating less and exercising more, try to increase lean muscle mass," writes physician Andrew Weil in his book *Healthy Aging: A Lifelong Guide to Your Well-Being*. Weight training, he said, will "keep the metabolic furnace burning bright."

I asked Bass about whether he ever thought of cutting back. What is the difference, I asked, between him and a 70-year-old man in excellent health who walks a little and putters in the yard?

"One thing he isn't trying to do is challenge or improve himself," Bass said. "It sounds like he's an old man, and that doesn't excite me. I think you have to find something that excites you, that motivates you, so you want to get out of the bed and get down to the gym."

AGING IS INEVITABLE

But Bass isn't bulletproof. There is the osteoarthritis in his lower back that has forced him to give up the use of his Concept2 rowing machine and traditional squats where the barbell rests behind the neck. He also has a weakness in his left shoulder and mild atrophy in his left triceps. On a visit to the Cooper Clinic, doctors discovered a buildup of calcium in his left anterior descending artery that requires the use of a statin drug to reduce cholesterol.

At 67, Bass also found out that he was retaining excessive amounts of urine in his bladder. After several tests, he had surgery to remove abnormal lobes where urine drains from the bladder through the prostate.

"The whole situation went against my experience so far and my optimistic view of the future," he wrote in *Great Expectations*. "I expected a few problems to come with aging, but frankly I didn't expect this so soon. I went to the doctor with what I considered a minor problem—and I ended up in surgery."

When he first met his urologist, the doctor had concluded that Bass would have to insert a device into his penis three or four times a day to keep the urinary pathway open. It seemed barbaric. Bass responded with understandable reluctance; later, after it was clear he would have to do something, Bass countered with using the device less. He has been able to pare down the number of sessions to once a week, with his doctor's blessing.

Then at 68, Bass had his right hip replaced. Neither Bass nor his doctors know why he needed the surgery, although hip replacements are the second-most common orthopedic surgery after knee replacements for people 65 to 84, according to a 2007 study by the federal Agency for Healthcare Research and Quality. Fifty years of weight training might have been the cause. Bass knows his share of old weightlifters who have had a hip replaced and who usually trace it back to an injury. "But I don't think that I would have gotten this far had I not been exercising," he said.

Rather than undergo a traditional hip replacement, he learned about an alternative procedure that causes less tissue damage because the hip is replaced through natural breaks in the muscle. His recovery was faster, although it left him with weakness in his hip flexor and numbness in his upper thigh. I noticed when we went for a walk, he moved stiffly at the beginning.

Bass's approach to aging underscores a trait I've seen in older superfit persons: They use knowledge, experience, and sometimes a healthy dose of independence to find a way to adapt.

Bass talked to me matter-of-factly about his ritual of keeping his urinary pathway open. The practice changed from dread to just another regimen in his life. He checked with knowledgeable friends and did his own research to find a better procedure for his hip replacement that was more fitting for his active lifestyle—even though it meant a trip to Houston for the surgery. He has dropped some exercises that cause problems for his body and added new ones. To get around weaknesses such as his osteoarthritis, he showed me how he clasped a belt around his waist that was attached to a biceps curl bar with weights. This way he could still do a squat and work his leg muscles while keeping pressure off his spine.

"One of the raps against older bodybuilders is that they are lean but they don't have any muscle—they don't have a butt," he said. "Believe me, I got a butt! I don't think that I am losing anything. I think that my butt is bigger than it was before."

For Bass, the hip replacement has become, in a sense, a badge of honor: The photo he used for his latest book is a softly lit nude that accentuated his signature abs and the surgical scar on the right hip.

Terry Todd said that Bass understands that his physique is more than a finely sculpted collection of muscle and bone. He and his photographs are playing a historic role, he said, in the fields of aging and popular culture. "I think that he has understood his role more clearly as the years have gone by," Todd said.

6

I Want to Be a Winner

I hadn't seen Philippa Raschker in more than a year when she emerged from a group of sprinters who had gathered at the end of the track. She was hobbling badly and I thought she had injured her Achilles tendon for the umpteenth time. Raschker, born in 1947, is the best women's age-group track athlete of all time. But for all her greatness, decades of running, jumping, and throwing have taken their toll. It seemed as if every superlative performance was followed by an injury.

It turned out she was fine. She went behind the stands at the Cardinal Park Track Stadium at the University of Louisville, and when she reappeared, I could see that she was stretching by walking on her heels. It's especially helpful for the Achilles but rarely used by older female athletes. I should have figured she had been doing something like this. Although there were a handful of other talented women over 50 who were competing in track events at the 2007 Summer National Senior Games, Raschker was in a class by herself.

She easily came in first in her preliminary heat of the 100-meter dash in a time of 13.97 seconds. It's a time that most men 20 years younger could not beat. I speak from experience. In my mid-40s, training five days a week, I was running only a few hundredths of a second faster.

During her introduction in the 100 to the several hundred people in the stands, the announcer had stumbled over her name. It's pronounced "Rash-ker." But during the 400-meter dash, he realized that she was in fact the star of the Games. The clock on the scoreboard flickered the time in seconds and hundredths of seconds as Raschker zoomed ahead of the field. By the time she was on the backstretch, he told the crowd that the runner in lane 7 had a chance to break the world record in her age group. As she sprinted the final 100 meters, many people in the stands rose to their feet and started shouting, clapping, and whistling for what was the most animated moment of the morning.

She finished in 1:08.54, missing the world record by a little more than a one second. (She would break it in 1:06.69 two days later in the finals.) The closest finisher was a 61-year-old runner from Michigan who had trailed her by nearly 22 seconds—more than the length of a football field.

Raschker had no idea she led by such a wide margin. She never heard the shouts from the crowd. She loves the limelight of the track and she understands that, in essence, she is performing for an audience. "But when I run and compete, I don't hear anything," she told me in Baton Rouge, Louisiana, in 2001 at the National Masters Track & Field Championships. "It's not that I am really concentrating so much; I'm blank. I go to the starting line with doubt. But once the gun goes off, everything goes on automatic and I run as fast as I can because I want to win. I want to be a winner."

Raschker has broken more than 200 U.S. and world records in nearly 30 years as an age-group competitor. Her greatest skill is her versatility. She competes in all of the sprint and field events, doing everything from running the 100-meter dash to throwing the javelin. Her only serious competition is at international meets, and thus, she spends much of her time training alone near her home in Marietta, Georgia, a suburb of Atlanta, for those rare moments on the world stage.

A BREED APART

Phil Raschker is 5-foot-4 and 110 pounds (162.5 cm, 50 kg). Her legs are chiseled from decades of track work; her biceps bulge from years of weight training and catapulting her body over the pole-vault bar. As with many great sprinters, her style is deceptive. She moves effortlessly down the track. Her head and torso are virtually motionless as her legs and arms drive forward. It is only when you watch her competing against other women her age—their faces contorted, so many movements wasted—that Raschker's true abilities shine.

At venues like the Senior Games, where one of the aims is merely to encourage people over 50 to exercise regularly, it could be easy to dismiss many of the others. But in fact, like Raschker, they are all outliers in a vast sea of inactivity as obesity in the United States has climbed steadily over the past two decades.

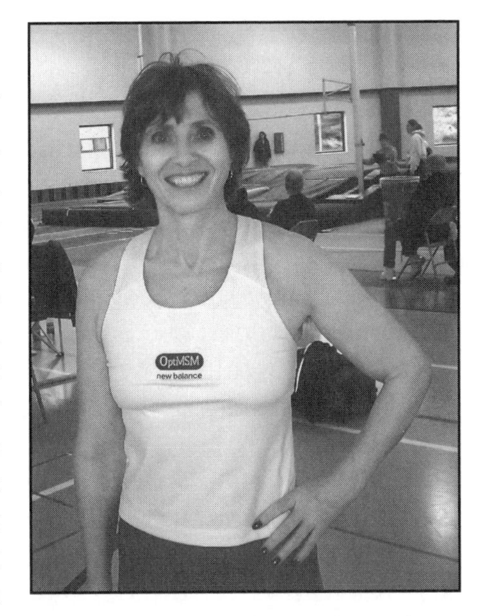

Philippa Raschker at a 2006 indoor meet at Carthage College in Kenosha, Wisconsin.

"We have a lot of people here whose skills are not even close to being elite," said Phil Godfrey, president and chief executive officer of the Senior Games Association. "And we love them just as much, if not more, than the elite-level athlete. Because that guy from Montana who can barely make it to the end of the pool in the 100-yard butterfly, and the only reason he got here is because he was the only guy from Montana to swim it in his state meet, he's going to go home and talk to his neighbors and tell them, 'That was so cool! You can't believe what happened to me in Louisville. Get in the water with me.' That's what it's all about: getting people involved and bringing somebody back."

Still, the Games and the sponsors hold up the hyperfit as role models. A photo of Raschker arching over the bar in the pole vault graced the front page of the 2007 Senior Games Web site.

"She is far and away the greatest masters athlete ever," said Tom Rauscher, then 61, a fellow pole vaulter from California.

Said Phil Mulkey, her former companion and a member of the U.S. Olympic track team in 1960, "There is nothing she lets stand in the way. Whether it is the fear of losing or the joy of winning—whatever it is—she's got it."

In 1995 at the U.S. Outdoor Championships, Raschker's third-place jump of 10 feet 10 inches (330 cm) in the pole vault at age 48, behind future Olympic gold medalist Stacy Dragila, was nominated by USA Track & Field as one of the top 25 moments in track over a quarter-century. In 1997 at age 50, she was recruited by Life University in Georgia for her prowess in the pole vault and multievents. Her time in the 200-meter dash that year was as fast as the best high school girls in Georgia. "The last thing you lose when you get older is your strength," said then-coach Mike Spino. "She's strong and she's fast and she's had a lot of experience." The school was a member of the National Association of Intercollegiate Athletics. The NAIA had no restrictions on age. But Raschker volunteered that she had received $300 for winning age-graded races at four meets over several years, jeopardizing her amateur status. The school asked that an exception be made, but the NAIA said no. There was a chance she could have joined the team the next year. But by then she had left school.

In 2003, Raschker became the oldest finalist for the James E. Sullivan Award as the nation's top amateur athlete. Other finalists were high school basketball star LeBron James, short-track speed skater Apolo Anton Ohno, guard Diana Taurasi of the University of Connecticut, and future record-breaking Olympic medalist Michael Phelps, who won.

Rauscher was part of a group that pushed the Amateur Athletic Union to nominate Raschker for the Sullivan Award. In Louisville, he had been helping her with her steps in the triple jump.

"She works hard at it," Rauscher said. "She doesn't train as hard as when she was younger—and that's good. But she is doing a lot. It's a combination of talent and work."

Raschker had brought an umbrella to shield her from the sun and a large bag with assorted shoes and warm-up gear. She was trying to finish the rest of her coffee as we walked to her awards ceremony for the triple jump—a block away from the track. It was 11:45 a.m. Raschker won't consume caffeine in the afternoon. In the auditorium, she rested a bag of ice on a tender foot as a precaution and watched the other presentations.

For some of the more than 12,000 athletes and their families, an awards ceremony at the Senior Olympics can be the crowning glory of a lifetime of sweat and toil. Raschker was in Louisville, essentially, to practice. Her next international meet would be in Italy, two months away, and her first in a new age bracket where she would presumably have the best chance to break new records and win more medals. As she stood on the podium, the stirring trumpets from John Williams's "Olympic Fanfare" filled the darkened auditorium. Six people were in the audience.

AN EARLY ATHLETE

Raschker was born in Hamburg, Germany. She grew up, in her eyes, an outcast. Her father was a British soldier whom she did not meet until years later. The other children in school had fathers, or they had been killed in the war. She made up stories about hers, cut out pictures of movie stars, and told classmates they were her father.

"I was angry," she told me. Her voice is surprisingly deep, like a smoker's, and she retains a strong German accent. "I thought it was my mother's fault. I took a lot of grief from the other kids."

She was raised by her mother and a woman who wasn't a relative but whom she called her aunt. It was her aunt who encouraged Raschker to play sports. She started at age 2 and took up track at 10. Sports were an outlet for what she perceived as ostracism from other children. She thinks that Germany's system of club teams laid a strong foundation because it exposed her to track and field, gymnastics, swimming, and other sports. She went to school through the ninth grade and completed an apprenticeship program in accounting.

At 20, she moved to the United States after breaking up with her boyfriend and worked as a governess for a German family in Washington, D.C. In her early years in the States, she joined a running club and ran in a few track meets. She had been invited to compete in a dual meet against Canadians, but a manager in an office where she had started working refused to give her the day off. "So I quit," she said.

She dabbled in bike racing for a few years but tired of it. She has a sprinter's personality and doesn't do well moving in low gear over long distances. "Cycling is like road racing—you just ride and ride and ride for practice," she said. "I am just not into distance. It doesn't do anything for me."

While living in North Carolina, she was leafing through the newspaper one day and saw the results of an age-group track meet. She had no idea there was such a thing. The next year, 1980, she started competing and winning right away. She was 33. "I just jumped in—I was so happy to do it," she said.

Raschker thinks that one of the reasons for her early success is that most women her age in the United States didn't have a background in track. It wasn't until 1975 that the first World Masters Track and Field Championships took place in Toronto. Of the 1,400 athletes entered, 80 were women. When Raschker first began competing in the pole vault, she was mostly going up against men. Her third-place finish in the pole vault at age 48 in 1995 was the first time it was held as an exhibition event for women in the Outdoor Track and Field National Championships.

Raschker was married for 10 years, divorced, never remarried, and never had children. In the 2004 documentary *Racing Against the Clock* about Raschker and four other older female track athletes, she described athletics as "my child, my family, my everything." Indeed, as a self-employed accountant working out of her home, she has been able to devote more time to training and traveling to track meets than many women. This ability to focus so much on the sport, combined with her talent, her ambition, and her relationship with Mulkey, has proven to be a lethal combination.

"The first time I saw her, I couldn't help but say something to her," he told me. "She was blessed with the ability to run as flawlessly in the sprints as any woman I've ever seen."

They lived and trained together in the Atlanta area for 18 years. Mulkey, an Olympic decathlete, was a specialist in the hurdles and pole vault. For years, they were often the best in their respective age groups in their events. In 1993, they were named the top masters athletes by USA Track and Field. They planned for major meets by reviewing videos of past performances that one of them shot of the other. Mulkey told me that he would sit in the stands with a telephoto lens and film Raschker; when they got home, they would use the footage to find ways to get better. Should she tweak the way she brought her trail leg over the hurdle? How could she adjust her stride to take full advantage of her short stature? What could be done to convert her speed down the runway of the pole vault into more power to lift herself over the bar? They would study the calendar of upcoming meets and coordinate Raschker's training schedule so she would peak at the right time and put her in the best possible position to break a record.

In the meets where I've seen her, she has won at will. But footage of the World Games that were shot in Puerto Rico in 2003 for *Racing Against the Clock* showed her gutting out 800 meters and collapsing at the finish with a spasm in her hamstring. She needed to finish the race to win the heptathlon. In another race, although her left hamstring was bandaged, she seemed to fly over the hurdles, edging another woman at the tape. Only after she crossed the line did she begin to limp badly.

The National Senior Games

The National Senior Games (www.nsga.com) are held every two years for men and women 50 and older. Competitors must first qualify by participating in NSGA-sanctioned state games. Generally, to earn a spot at the national games, competitors must be among the top three finishers in an event or earn a qualifying time.

Featured medal sports are archery, badminton, basketball, bowling, cycling (5K and 10K time trials and 20K and 40K road races), golf, horseshoes, racewalk (1,500-meter and 5K), racquetball, road race (5K and 10K), shuffleboard, softball, swimming, table tennis, tennis, track and field, triathlon, and volleyball.

Demonstration sports are equestrian, fencing, lawn bowling, rowing, sailing, soccer, and water polo.

The games began in 1987 in St. Louis and drew 2,500 athletes. In 2009, 12,750 athletes are expected to compete (www.2009seniorgames.org). The next two games are in Houston in 2011 and in Cleveland in 2013.

"Oh, God, I was afraid of those hurdles," she said as the camera shows her getting a massage under a tent. "That's all right, as long as I can triple-jump tomorrow."

"Ah, you won't be triple-jumping tomorrow," someone in the tent told her.

"I am jumping tomorrow!" she said, her voice rising. "I told you until they scrape me off of the floor, I'm going to compete."

UNDER AN OLYMPIAN'S TUTELAGE

"Drive," Mulkey told me, "that's the big thing. That's the biggest difference with her—she just can't stand losing. Can't stand it."

Raschker and Mulkey would often make a game of it during their workouts. In the beginning, Mulkey would spot her a foot in the long jump, but over time the games became more competitive. "At first, I looked like a frog," she said. "But then I learned to get my legs out in front of me and get my butt dirty."

"At first," Mulkey said, "when we would train together in the 200 meters, I would run the outside lane, virtually patting her on the butt, 'Keep up, keep up, keep up.' It wasn't long after that—she was patting me on the butt and saying, 'Keep up, keep up, keep up.'"

Mulkey, 14 years older than Raschker, still had great technique but was losing speed. Meanwhile, Raschker was still learning events and making improvements. "Over the years, I would get a little better and he would get a little older," she said. "It made the training fun." In fact, Mulkey was providing invaluable advice. "He was a perfectionist," she said. "In a sense it was the key to my becoming athletically who I became because I really don't think that, had I been on my own, I would have trained so hard." She still marvels at Mulkey's ability to spot flaws and correct them. Mulkey could see something in another athlete he admired and imitate it almost immediately. "What a gift," she said. "For me it was repetition."

Not that these sessions always went smoothly. Raschker told me that Mulkey could be impatient. He didn't always understand why she didn't pick up something faster.

Mulkey moved to Birmingham, Alabama, in 2000, and when we talked in September 2007 he was 74 and working as an assistant track coach at a private high school. "She is not easy to coach," he said. "She is very sensitive and very headstrong, but that plays into athletic ability. Somehow we got together and she realized that we would be of value to one another." The two of them still visit and talk by phone or send e-mail regularly. Mulkey told me that he still loved her.

Raschker is so focused on what she is doing that when she talks about past world meets, and the injuries that seem to intertwine them, she assumes it's common knowledge. Her preoccupation with track, combined with all of the advances in off-the-shelf accounting software, has eaten into her business. "She made a decision some time ago that she was going to do the track and field game and worry about work second," said Mulkey, a retired businessman.

Raschker lives frugally and seldom goes out. She rents out part of her house to cut expenses. "Basically, I make my choices," she told me in the winter of 2006 at a track meet at Carthage College in Kenosha, Wisconsin. "I think that I eat well enough—last night I had steak. I don't think that I deprive myself. I don't really feel as if I'm missing anything. It's a state of mind, really, for what makes us happy."

Raschker spends upwards of $10,000 a year on the sport, much of it for traveling to meets. She was getting ready to buy an elliptical trainer when we met at Carthage because it's easier on the body. Earlier, she had purchased a stationary recumbent bike for the same reason. She lifts weights in an unheated space under her kitchen porch. She runs at a high school track a few miles from home.

Because she participates in so many events, Raschker can seem to be everywhere at track meets, treating the oval and the infield as her stage. One minute she's running the hurdles. Then it's off to the high-jump pit. Then she has to collect a medal. She will often appear nervous and preoccupied. Other times she'll chat up fellow athletes or run into the stands to talk with friends. Over the years, I have found her to be self-absorbed but amiable and compassionate as well. Unlike many masters athletes I've interviewed, she asked me about my job and my family. At Baton Rouge, she jogged over to sit down with Pat Peterson, a sprint specialist who was then 75 years old. Peterson was entered to run but has not yet fully recovered from a near-death experience with non-Hodgkin's lymphoma. Raschker had sent her batches of cards when she was in the hospital, with a note asking her to open a new card every day.

"For whatever reason, I feel very comfortable in this milieu," she said. "I certainly grew up not bragging about myself, or stepping forward and saying, 'Hey, I'm an athlete and this is what I can do.'"

But with the rest of her life, she has less confidence, "though I'm getting a lot better," she said. At a party, especially if she doesn't know a lot of people, "I love to just sit in the corner and watch it all. Drink it in. Listen to everybody. You won't find me making conversation. I am very intimidated by that."

"Phil is an open book," said Liz Johnson, a friend from Charlotte, North Carolina, who took up sprinting when she was 40 and competes in multievents with Raschker. "She really does have low self-esteem—she competes for a reason."

Raschker told me once that her best year was 1997 when she was 50 years old and won 10 gold medals at an international meet, the World Masters Championships in Durban, South Africa.

Since then, she has struggled with a series of injuries: She has had surgery on her Achilles; her knees have been operated on three times; she's been plagued by lower-back pain and a chronically sore left hamstring. She retired briefly in 1998, fed up with internal politics of masters track, and as she told Ken Stone, a journalist and the blogger of masterstrack.com, "Too many meets, too many events, too many years. I'm tired."

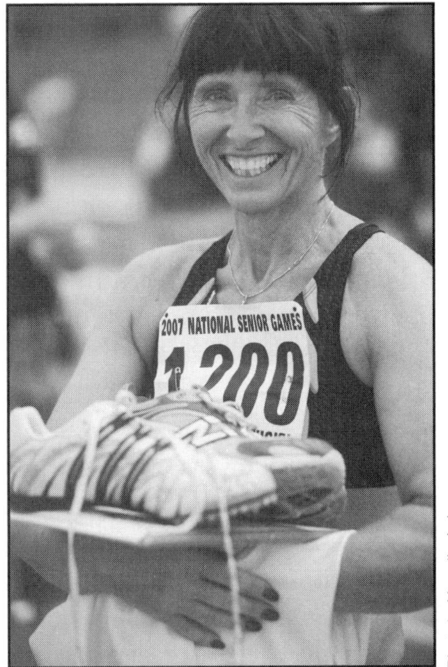

Photo by Veronika Lukasova

Philippa Raschker in 2007, the year she eased back on training to help avoid injury.

Raschker is bothered by the fact that she began accumulating small amounts of cellulite on her legs in her 50s. "Other people say, 'Hey, you have a great-looking body,'" she told me. "But I just plain don't like to be this way." This small consequence of aging is part of a larger struggle. How could Raschker continue building her résumé as the most dominant female age-group track athlete?

"Basically, I want to stay as close as possible to the previous year's performances," she said. "But I am realistic and I know that it's not possible. You don't fall off every year. It occurs every two or three years, and then you go down. Your times are not as fast as they were. Your jumps are not as high as they once were. It keeps coming, in chunks."

To contend with these inevitabilities, Raschker has had to make adjustments and overcome injuries. It's required new training methods. She's had to measure her performances differently. And to keep her competitive fire burning, she has had to search for new ways to motivate herself.

One of the things that pulled her out of her retirement was when the maker of the nutritional supplement CustomVite offered to sponsor her. "I had tried for years and years to get a sponsor and I never got anywhere," she said. "So when they approached me, that gave me an added incentive and I wanted to do well." After four years, she moved to another supplement company that made OptiMSM, a sulfur-based nutritional compound. She's looked for other sponsorships, but in vain.

In 2003, she took off four months in the hope that her aching hamstring would heal. She was getting ultrasound and chiropractic treatment before she left for the inaugural World Masters Indoor Championships in Sindelfingen, Germany. The doctors weren't sure what her problem was—her back, knee, and hamstring were all hurting.

The rest hadn't helped. In her first race, the 200 meters, she re-injured the hamstring. All of the money for rehab and travel, and now she had to sit out most events. "My brain just started racing at that point," she said. She gambled and tried the high jump and won her only gold medal. It was her worst performance ever at a world championship. When she returned home, she told me that she didn't know what she was going to do. She felt she was capable of great performances in the years ahead—if only her body would cooperate.

"I need to step away from it," she said. "I can't train right now. I need to look at the cost of this. It's extremely expensive as a hobby. It gets frustrating and you train very hard and you want to see what you can do, and you are sidelined almost immediately. At this point I don't feel as if I am holding up that well anymore. I am going to have to reevaluate the whole thing. Maybe it's time to do fewer events."

Sindelfingen was instructive. She began to see that she was going to have to ease off in her training, especially the pounding of the track, until a meet drew closer. She would have to rely more on her recumbent bike and elliptical trainer. When we met at Carthage, she had replaced much of her speed work with hard running three days a week on a treadmill, dialing up the speed by 0.1 mile an hour every week or so. Her goal was to rest and heal up for 2007, when she turned 60.

"If it doesn't work, I'm going to look at the whole situation and decide what to do," she said. "I enjoy being fit, so I need to find something to get fit—to give me a goal to put out there. I might want to try . . ." she looked at me blankly. "I can't remember in English—that thing on the water."

"Rowing?"

"Yeah, rowing, because I have good upper-body strength and even though my knees aren't the strongest, I can fold them up enough and there's not so much impact."

By her own admission, Raschker is having memory problems. Though she seemed to have strong recall of most of the questions I asked, she told me, "I don't remember stuff. I've always had memory problems, but as I age, it seems to get worse. At work, account numbers I have used for 30 years—I get a blank. It's totally gone. It's those kinds of things that totally scare me."

This could be a natural part of aging, or menopause, since scientists have been exploring the relationship between forgetfulness and a drop in estrogen levels. I've noticed occasional blips in my own memory in my 50s, and so do others around me. Is it a problem? Or as an athlete who is acutely aware of her physical decline, is Raschker more attuned to the aging process than many of us?

Liz Johnson thinks Raschker's memory problem needs more attention. "Have I seen a change in her?" she asked. "Yes, I can see a change," she said. "She needs to get more information and see what she can do about it."

Another impetus for Raschker, and all age-group athletes, is the allure of entering a new age group, where the marks, invariably, are slightly lower, the times slightly slower. It's an opportunity to start over, so to speak. That's what Raschker was doing in 2007. Also, track statisticians have devised a tool called age-graded tables that measure performances against the marks of athletes of other ages. In this way, as Raschker has aged and ebbed, she has been able to plug in a mark and compare it to women in open events who are in their 20s and 30s. According to one of these tables, Raschker's 13.92 seconds in the 100 at age 60 was equivalent to a 10.78 in open competition. At the age of 50, her 12.5 was worth 10.69. (The world record for elites is Florence Griffith-Joyner's 10.49 in 1988.)

Age-Graded Tables

Age-graded tables, produced by World Masters Athletics (WMA), are a tool used for comparing performances. They allow older athletes to "convert" their marks to those made in open competitions (for ages 20 to 30.) For example, a 64-year-old male who runs the 100-meter dash in 15 seconds would learn his time corresponds to 12.25 seconds in open competition. An online calculator by British professor Howard Grubb employs the WMA tables. Grubb's calculator can be found at www.howardgrubb.co.uk/athletics/wmalookup06.html.

The tables allow athletes to compare their performances with other athletes regardless of age or sex. This is often done at track meets and road races to determine an age-graded winner. The same man who ran 15 second in the 100 would have an age-graded percentage of 79.92 percent. WMA says any mark higher than 90 percent is considered world class. Any mark over 80 percent is national class. Over 70 percent is regional class, and over 60 percent is local class.

The tables have other uses: to compare a mark with those of previous years, to compare performances in different events, or to allow an athlete to set goals for the future.

"I want to know where I am year by year," she said. "Age grading allows me to compare my performance regardless of age. I feel I can improve by working on my technique because physically our bodies deteriorate as we age. We are not going to run as fast or jump as high. But we can hold our own longer because of technique."

A strict age-graded comparison of Raschker's time in the 100 reveals a slight drop over the past decade. But Raschker's true strength is in multi-events, where a combination of speed, strength, and endurance is needed. In June 2007, she broke the world record in the seven-event heptathlon—her specialty—by scoring 6,865 points at the National Masters Heptathlon

How She Did It: At 60, Philippa Raschker Wins Gold

Raschker won 10 gold medals at the 17th World Masters Athletics Outdoor Track and Field Championships in Riccione, Italy, in September 2007.

Later that year, Raschker was named Female World Masters Athlete of the Year by World Masters Athletics Association for her performances in Riccione and at other meets during the year. She set a total of 12 world records in 2007. (In 2008, she had another great year and was named USA Track & Field Masters Athlete of the Year and was again a finalist for the Sullivan Award.)

She attributed the record to cutting back and doing her easiest workouts ever:

- She eliminated jumps and hurdles from her training altogether—except for a day or two before a meet.
- She ran every other day and either lifted weights or ran on her elliptical trainer the other days. The elliptical trainer kept her aerobically strong but did not put undue stress on joints and muscles.
- On some days, she did nothing at all.

She no longer ran sprints as fast as she could in practice:

- She ran slower—about 85 percent of the age-group world-record time.
- After warming up, she would pick a distance—100, 150, 200, or 300 meters. She would run 10 sprints at that distance.
- Each distance required a different rest period: 3 minutes after each 100, 5 minutes after each 150, 7 minutes after each 200, and 10 minutes after each 300.

Championships in Hoover, Alabama. Athletes are awarded points based on how fast they run, how high they jump, and how far they throw the shot and the javelin. For age-group athletes, software converts an athlete's performance to the marks of athletes in open competition. The data are then plugged into a table devised by the world governing body for track and field to determine the total points. Raschker's point total was higher than her world-record totals at ages 50 and 55. She broke the old age-group record for women 60 to 64 by nearly 1,000 points.

Raschker was buoyant. She had broken the world heptathlon record in Alabama; then in Louisville, she had broken the record for the 400-meter dash. Next was the World Masters Athletics Outdoor Track and Field Championships in the resort city of Riccione, Italy, in September 2007.

I didn't see any of this on TV and didn't expect to. Television covers little track these days and ignores masters sports entirely. But I read accounts from Ken Stone, who was busy tracking events from San Diego, and I caught glimpses of Raschker and others on YouTube. In all, Raschker competed in 22 events in an exhausting 12 days. Taken in their entirety, what I saw from these men and women was a time line of the possibilities of the human body as we age.

In Riccione, Raschker won 10 gold medals, placing first in nine individual events and dropping down to the 55-to-59 age group to win a 10th gold in the 4 × 100 relay. With a slight but legal tailwind, she broke the world age-group record for the 80-meter hurdles in a time of 13.26 seconds.

"Basically, I am injury free," she told me before she left for Italy. "We all have aches and pains, but I feel really—I haven't felt this good in years. I've been reborn. I love it. I can go to the track and do the things that I want to do."

7

A Runner's Heart

Greg Osterman was among the hordes of runners waiting in the darkness for the start of the 2005 Flying Pig Marathon in downtown Cincinnati, Ohio. Those who couldn't keep a lid on their energy found little patches of space in which to jog. Some looked as if they were rushing off to work as they slurped down bowls of cereal and jabbered on their cell phones. Others took last sips of coffee and energy drinks and stared blankly at the spectacle around them. Osterman was leaning against a lamppost. It was spring, and even though he had spent much of the year jogging indoors on a treadmill, he was deeply tanned. His gray hair was flecked with silver; his mustache was white as bone china. When we met up, his affable manner had evaporated. It was clear his mind was in another place. His face—like rawhide—was impassive, and maybe because he used to smoke I couldn't help but think he looked like the Marlboro Man in running shorts.

Osterman, 50, had a fitful night of sleep and was still shaking the cobwebs out of his head. He said little. He is not talkative by nature. But when it comes to his heart transplant and the cancer that followed, he seemed to almost relish explaining how his world had been slipping away before a teenage girl's heart, and later, running, turned his life around.

A SURVIVOR

The scene along the Ohio River was beginning to brighten with the first signs of dawn. A warm, red glow burned into the horizon, and moments later, the sun crested over the hills in Kentucky. As if on cue, the crowd's mood changed: Jackets were tossed away. Spouses were kissed and babies were returned to their strollers. There were handshakes all around. The Rolling Stones' "Start Me Up" kick-started from giant speakers. The crowd swelled from sidewalks and the grass and poured into the street as Osterman was swallowed by the mosh pit of expectant runners. The starter counted down the seconds, followed by a loud boom. The runners and onlookers cheered and a great movement of legs and lungs and Lycra surged forward as thousands of hearts began beating faster and faster.

All except Osterman's. He poked along at a slow jog for some 3 miles (5 km) before he started to get into his groove. He does this every time he runs. He starts slowly, allowing time for a pair of naturally occurring hormones to go to work and get his heart beating fast enough—about 130 beats a minute—to meet the demands of long-distance running. If he took off like a shot, his heart would go into overdrive. He could pass out. He doesn't wear a heart-rate monitor; instead he jogs easily until he feels he is ready to push harder. "It's more a matter of feel," he told me as we were meeting with his cardiologist.

"His messaging system is completely gone," said Dr. Lynne Wagoner. "When you get ready to exercise, your brain tells your heart that you are going to exercise. Almost immediately if you go on a treadmill your heart rate will go up in anticipation of exercise. In other words, there is a connection between your brain and your muscles and your heart."

When Osterman had his transplant in October 1992 at 37, doctors had to cut the nerves that bounce signals between the brain and the heart. A transplant recipient depends on slower-moving hormones, epinephrine and norepinephrine, to send messages to the brain, signaling it's time for the heart to beat faster.

Osterman and I had wandered through the labyrinth of hallways of the hospital at the University of Cincinnati until we found Wagoner's office. The two of them hugged. Osterman was once a regular. But as his health improved, he stops by only every six months for check-ups, which include a heart biopsy—a procedure where a tube is fed down a vein in his neck and a piece of tissue is taken to make sure his body is not rejecting it. He's greeted fondly—like a former student who's done well for himself. He's beaten the odds and outlived most others who had transplants in the early 1990s. In the past decade there have been 2,000 to 2,300 heart-transplant procedures per year in the United States, according to data supplied by the United Network for Organ Sharing. At the time of his visit with Dr. Wagoner, about 52 percent of the people who had heart transplants the same year as Osterman were dead, according to UNOS.

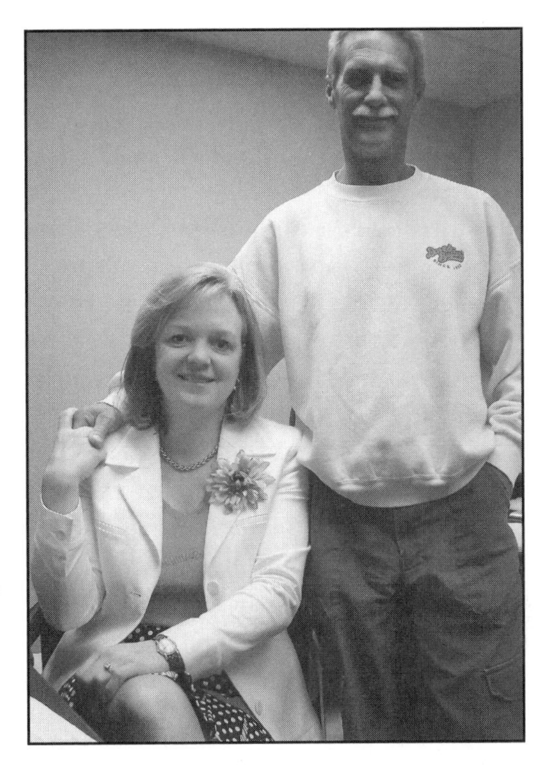

Greg Osterman and Lynne Wagoner, his cardiologist.

Five years after he got a new heart, Osterman ran his first marathon. He has run a total of six marathons. At first, Dr. Wagoner had her reservations. No one was sure if any heart transplant recipient had ever run a marathon before. "I didn't know whether it was particularly good for a transplanted heart," she said. "I have always been a proponent of exercise. I just had no idea what 26 miles would do."

There were not only questions about his heart. Doctors wondered whether his skeletal system could withstand the miles of pounding. But working in his favor was the fact that he had stopped taking prednisone, an anti-inflammatory drug that can make bones more brittle. Also, his new heart was a better match than most donor hearts, and he hadn't backslid into a lifestyle of unhealthy habits. Consequently, doctors were able to wean him off drugs that were both life sustaining and debilitating. He takes only three pills to control blood pressure and the antirejection medicine he will take the rest of his life. His emotional state was better than most transplant recipients, too. "Many patients tend to use having a heart transplant as a crutch: They tend to dwell on it," Wagoner said. "With younger patients, the ones who are about 20, they tend to reach a point where they think they don't need the medicines anymore. A lot of it is self-discipline."

Osterman had been sitting quietly. He seemed unaware that the odds of living this long were nearly 50–50, but Dr. Wagoner also said the hospital had a handful of patients who have lived close to 20 years after transplants. "That's good to know," he said, offering a weak smile. He told us that he used to go to a support group for people with new hearts. "I shouldn't say this, but I felt out of place," he said.

She nodded. "A lot of them, they tend to focus on the negative and the problems they are experiencing," she said. "Most patients, I think, because they can't get back to what was normal before, they just don't even make much of an effort. We send all of them to cardiac rehab and try to get all of them back to some kind of physical conditioning, but most don't. I think that Greg's unique because much of what he's accomplished is with willpower."

After we left Dr. Wagoner's office, we passed through the wreckage of upended lives. People in pajamas shuffled through the hallway tethered to tubes of dripping medicine. Others were being pushed in wheelchairs or lying atop gurneys. These were people who may have been dealt a bad genetic hand, but some had been pushing their odds for years with cigarettes, poor diets, and little exercise. I was anxious to get outside and Osterman was, too.

"Something clicks when you are 50," he said. "You aren't going to live forever. You only have so much time. My life is so different from my dad—he smoked one to two packs of Camel straights a day. By the time he was 50, he was shot. I spent all of those years watching him going downhill. It was just a long, slow deterioration. It was hard to watch."

Osterman's own descent was quicker. It began with flu-like symptoms—tightness in his chest and a lack of energy. Osterman, then 36 and a plumber, could barely make it through the day. An echocardiogram revealed he had an enlarged heart. His cardiologist said he had contracted a viral infection that had attacked the heart muscles, sharply reducing his heart's ability to pump blood. The heart was also leaking blood. "He told me point blank, 'You've got problems,'" Osterman recalled. "'You are going to have to change your lifestyle. You are no longer going to be a plumber. The most you are going to be able to do is sit at home and maybe plant a few flowers.'"

Cardiomyopathy is a chronic disease that eventually leads to heart failure. Today, drugs can sustain a patient longer. But in 1990 when Osterman first got sick, drugs were less effective. By the fall of 1991, his medication had stopped working.

Jim Vanden Eynden is one of Osterman's oldest friends. He remembered a party when the hard-drinking Osterman told friends how sick he really was. "He was drinking nonalcoholic beer," he said. "He was totally gray. He looked bad. He had been telling us he didn't have any energy, but nobody knew [in] how bad of shape he was."

Osterman had to quit his job. Then he got into a car accident, and grudgingly, he agreed to quit driving. He couldn't balance his checkbook. He stayed in bed most of the time. His trips to the hospital were becoming more and more frequent. The prospect of dying was so palpable that he was having panic attacks and he had to go to a psychiatrist. He needed a new heart, but doctors told him he wasn't sick enough yet. "They told me you have to be on death row to get a transplant," he said.

These are all details he has gleaned over time from his doctors and his family. At the time, "For me, everything was pretty much a blank," he recalled.

A PICTURE OF HEALTH

Osterman lives in Loveland, a suburb of Cincinnati, in an immaculate split-level home. The ceiling of the living room reaches two stories and looks out on his backyard. The grass was lush from recent rains, and Osterman was itching to mow it. We were sitting in his kitchen and he drank from a bottle of water ("Hydrating," he said, for the Flying Pig). For the next two days, he would almost always have a bottle of water in his hand. It dawned on me: Carrying the water, his impressive physique, his tan (touched up at a tanning parlor), and certainly his running were all part of his persona. Osterman wants the world to know he is a very healthy man.

His wife, Carole, walked into the kitchen. She is warm, sunny, and outgoing. It's hard to imagine a time when the world was crumbling around her. As her husband was dying, she was holding down a part-time job with a florist and raising their two sons, Jason, who was then nine, and Danny, who was seven. "We just kind of existed," she said. "We just kind of lived day to day. I never looked past the next day."

Greg repeated what he had told me several times: "Carole had the worst of it," he said. "I was not functioning. I knew in my mind I was getting worse and worse. I would tell Carole that I didn't want to be here in the house because I thought I was going to go, I was going to die."

Then his father died. Osterman has no recollection of it. He was too sick to go to the funeral.

Greg's donor, he would learn, was an 18-year-old woman who had been killed in a crash near Dayton, Ohio. On October 26, 1992, Carole got a call from the hospital. "They called to say that they had a donor heart and that (Greg) was on the way to UC hospital for the surgery," she recalled. "I was in shock. I walked into the backyard. A neighbor was there and I told him, 'Greg's going to get a new heart.' He didn't know what to say to me—we just looked at each other."

Afterward he was on a respirator, and for three days Carole was at his bedside trying to get him to wake up and breathe on his own.

"When I came to, it was like, 'Wow!' It was something strange," he said. "You are aware of everything. I knew where I was. I knew who the people were. It was an instant feeling of being better. Everything was working again." He left the hospital after 14 days. At home, he walked to the grocery store and carried home jugs of milk to build up his strength. He was so weak Carole kidded him that he teetered on his walks like Charlie Chaplin.

But then his weakened condition conspired against him. Three months after the transplant, he was diagnosed with non-Hodgkin's lymphoma, a rare outcome of transplant surgery. He underwent more surgery. This time it was to remove 18 inches of small intestine and 12 inches of large intestine, his gall bladder, and part of his colon. Osterman tried getting healthy again as doctors struggled to find the right balance of medications to fight rejection and ward off a new invasion of cancer cells. He spent much of the next year on disability. Insurance and Medicaid paid for nearly all of the $500,000 in medical bills.

Osterman also struggled emotionally. He was taking up to 30 pills a day—a constant reminder he wasn't out of the woods. His heart had failed him. Then he got cancer. What would happen next?

Life is a series of altered expectations and how we respond to setbacks can be defining moments in our lives. Osterman desperately wanted to be healthy again. He attacked his recovery with a vengeance. He listened to what his doctors were telling him. He drank grape juice by the gallons. He ate egg whites and lots of fruits and vegetables. After spending so long depending on others, he wanted to be able to support his family again. He longed to get back to work. The hard, dirty work of installing plumbing on construction sites would validate his recovery well before he thought of running a marathon.

After high school, "Greg was going through jobs all of the time," Vanden Eynden recalled. "But when he got into plumbing, he found something he really liked."

Exercise became a means to an end. He loved being part of a crew that started with dirt and turned it into buildings. He wanted to make sure that if he returned, he could carry his load. "I knew that if I wanted to get back into it, I had a long way to go," Osterman said. "That's really why I started pushing myself to get back into that lifestyle—because that's all I knew." Three years after his heart transplant, at 40, he went back to work.

Walking had become a key to his recovery, and one day he suddenly broke into a slow jog. "I didn't even know if I could run," he said. "I picked it up a little bit and said to myself, 'Man, this doesn't feel too bad, and I don't feel too bad. I think everything is working. Let's try keeping this going and see how everything goes.'" He could feel his heart pounding—it was working. "It gave me a sense of well-being," he said. "This thing is really pumping and I'm feeling really good. I just wanted to keep it going."

In March 1994, there was a fund-raiser called the Heart Mini-Marathon, and he set his sights on being in it. As it drew closer, his exercise regimen was going so well that he decided to run the 5K in the morning and walk 6 miles with Carole in the afternoon.

"When he told us that he was going to run, we said, 'You're nuts,'" said Vanden Eynden. "'You're lucky to be alive.'"

His medical team was also apprehensive. "They told me if I started to get light-headed, I had to stop," he said. "They said it was just like the throttle on your car: If I started it too fast, I would stall. It kind of gave me a scare." He started slowly—about 11 minutes a mile—and ended at a jogger's pace of 9 minutes and 30 seconds a mile.

"When I finished, it gave me a shot of confidence that you couldn't believe," he said. "When someone tears into you and starts pulling things out of you, and then they say, 'OK, you are OK to go,' you just don't know if you are or not. It was a big shot in the arm. Everything the doctors were doing, and all of the work I was doing, it all came together. It told me I could move on."

He also started thinking about running a marathon. He had never been a jogger. He knew nothing about the aerobic world—to run simply for the joy of running. Construction work had been his exercise. At 5-feet-8 and 170 pounds (173 cm, 77 kg), he was built more like a shortstop than a runner.

"The remarkable achievement about Greg is that he hadn't done any of this stuff before," said Les Potapczyk, a marathoner from Niagara Falls, Ontario, he met through running. "Greg wasn't a runner. For him to have an almost revelation, to say, 'I have to do something to keep me going,' to me, that's just phenomenal."

"When I first started running," Osterman said, "it was kind of a challenge. I went out real slow—5Ks, 10Ks—and then I got to a point that I could do those fairly easily. I thought that maybe with a little help I could stretch this out to a marathon."

He joined Team in Training, a program of the Leukemia & Lymphoma Society for aspiring citizen athletes. TNT uses coaches and mentors so participants can run or walk a marathon or half marathon, complete a triathlon, or cycle a 100-mile bike ride. TNT has the double-barreled effect of helping people achieve their goal of knocking off a significant aerobic milestone while helping collect donations.

Osterman's group ran once during the week and again on Saturday mornings. "He was always a little antsy and that made me worry about him," recalled Charlene Doran, a TNT mentor who had started running only a year and a half earlier. Osterman can get restless, chafing to cut the lawn, for example, and he's perpetually early for appointments. "Sometimes he was so anxious to get going that he would take off before some of the other runners had even gotten there," Doran said.

TNT offered the help he needed. He was getting coaching and tips on nutrition, injuries, and race strategy. Over a span of five months, he followed a plan to ramp up his training runs to 10 miles, then 15 miles, and finally, 20 miles (16, 24, and 32 km).

"Greg was not a naturally gifted runner," Doran said. "In the beginning, he would wear himself out. But he was competitive and he learned to pace himself."

Karen Cosgrove, the head coach of the TNT program in Cincinnati, remembered how Osterman's name jumped out on forms of runners' names she was reading.

"By the time he came into the program, there were 150 to 200 people doing it at any one time," Cosgrove said. "You become a number. So I had this program set up where you had to fill out this questionnaire and there was this question, 'Tell me about yourself. Are there any physical things we should be aware of?' People would tell us about their bad backs, their right ankle bothers them a little bit. Their muscles are tight. Then I come across Greg's: 'I just recovered from a heart transplant.'"

Cosgrove immediately called her sister, a nurse, and calls were made to Osterman's doctors. Everyone agreed that if he took it easy, it was OK for him to run.

The connection with TNT was fortuitous. Doran became a friend and running buddy. With Cosgrove, Osterman could draw on the expertise of a marathoner who had qualified for the Olympic Trials in 1984 and 1988 and had run 50 marathons.

"There is so much up and down to running a marathon—it's like life," Cosgrove said. "That's what I kept telling him. You are going to have peaks and valleys going through this race. The peaks: Enjoy. The valleys: Just know that you have the strength and the courage and don't be afraid to rise above it."

In January 1998, Osterman and Cosgrove entered the Bermuda Marathon. A warm sun occasionally burned through the clouds. But much of the race was cool, windy, and rainy. Cosgrove ferried water and gave encouragement as she moved between Osterman and another runner from Cincinnati. Osterman struggled at times. But Cosgrove kept telling him that he had done his homework. "This was the icing on the cake. The pain, the self-doubt, and getting past all that are what make marathoning so rewarding," she told him. "The irony is that he probably inspired me more than I inspired him."

Osterman and Cosgrove finished together at 5:01:23. Carole, sons Jason and Danny, and Osterman's mother were at the finish line.

"I can't tell you what it did for me," he said as we drove through Cincinnati traffic to pick up his bib and race packet for the Flying Pig. "It put everything in its spot. It was something that I thought I would never do. It was something for me to prove. 'If I can do this,' I thought, 'look what it says for this operation.' It works."

Later that year, he ran his second marathon in San Diego. The next year he ran the New York City Marathon and his first of three Flying Pigs. Heart transplant recipients who run marathons are rare, and there may be no one in the world who has run as many.

MEDICAL ADVANCES

Osterman's achievements underscore the advances in transplant medicine and the ability of some recipients to resume not only normal lives, but astonishingly active lives. The first heart transplant recipient, Louis Washkansky, was 55 and lived for 18 days after South African surgeon Christiaan Barnard transplanted a young woman's heart in 1967. The first transplant Olympics took place in 1978 in Great Britain when Maurice Slapak, a transplant surgeon, brought together about 100 kidney transplant recipients. More than 1,500 athletes who were transplant recipients participated in the 2007 World Transplant Games in Bangkok, Thailand, according to the organizers.

Osterman is healthier than most men his age. And perhaps because he is so robust, he flirts ever so slightly with the old days. Vanden Eynden, his best friend, told me how Osterman "would work all day, and then maybe he'd go sit in the bar. That was his routine." Now he might surprise a table of friends at a restaurant by ordering a shot of tequila. Two nights before the Flying Pig, we were together at a reception for the race as he wolfed down hors d'oeuvres and drank several beers. But these are blips. The transplant and the running "totally turned him around," Vanden Eynden said. "He's still Greg, but he is ambitious."

His doctors don't believe that his younger heart gives him any physical advantages. His engine might have fewer miles than other men his age, but he's not a race car. During our visit, Dr.

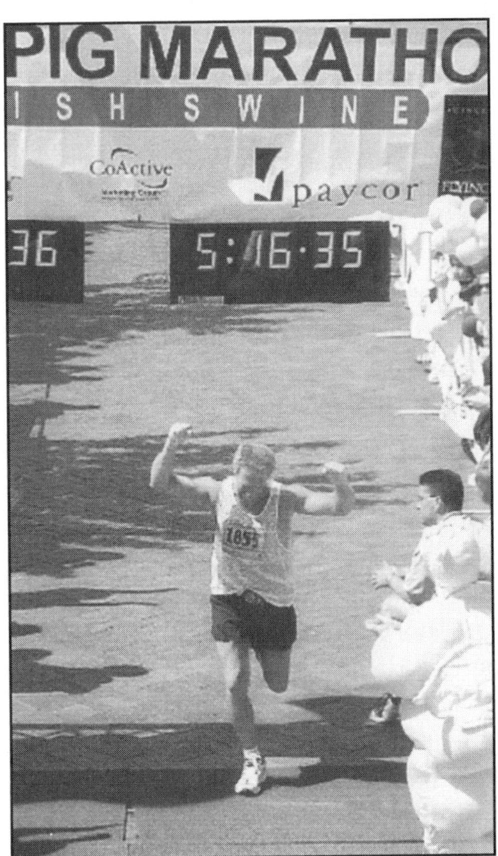

runphotos.com

Crossing a finish line is a confirmation to Greg Osterman that his health remains strong.

Wagoner scanned through Osterman's file and noted the results of a stress test after his first marathon in 1998 showed that his heart had performed at the capacity of an average man his age—100 percent of normal. A nurse in her office who was running the 2005 Flying Pig registered 160 percent of normal. Most heart transplant recipients perform at 50 to 60 percent of normal.

Osterman's heart rate in the stress test increased to 145 beats per minute after eight minutes of exercise. A normal heart, she said, would have been beating faster and reached that point more quickly with the help of nerves that Osterman lost from the surgery. "The lack of nerve input from the brain usually causes a person with a transplanted heart to wear out quickly when he exercises," Dr. Wagoner said. "The ability to sustain exercise for a long time is rare." Dr. Wagoner thinks Osterman has trained his heart to remain within a range of relative comfort for a long time. "It's become mind over matter," she said.

As terrible as it all was, the transplant and the cancer were the best things that ever happened to him. He lives a healthier life and believes he would never be in the shape he is now had he not gotten a new heart. The universe of marathon-running, cancer-surviving heart transplant recipients is tiny, and it's afforded him a status that would not have come his way. His recovery opened up his world and allowed him to touch the lives of others. He was the official spokesperson for the Flying Pig for several years. In Niagara Falls, Ontario, he shared his story on a podium with marathon great Dick Beardsley, a frequent speaker on the running circuit who was nearly killed in a farm accident and overcame a subsequent addiction to painkillers. Osterman was invited to run in California with Dean Karnazes, author of *Ultramarathon Man: Confessions of an All-Night Runner*, and received a mention in the book.

As we were walking to pick up his race credentials, Osterman was stopped a few times by admirers. "I think what you are doing is great," said one woman. A local TV anchor said hello (the station had done a story on him). The Cincinnati papers have written numerous articles on him. He was profiled by *Runner's World* in 2003.

Osterman even used a publicist to help drum up speaking engagements and find sponsors to pay for him to go to races. His message was simple: He recounts his journey from death's door to marathon runner, and he encourages others to overcome adversity, set goals, and meet them.

"Inspiration, heroism, role model—that's what we need as human beings," Potapczyk said. "If that helps you get inspired, or gets you through a personal crisis, then Greg's done his job."

One of Osterman's first motivational talks was to students at an elementary school in Cincinnati. "Underachievers," he described them. He recounted details of the surgery and his slow recovery. He didn't push a button, or wake up one day and suddenly start feeling better. It took hard work and the help of others to make him believe he could return to work and run marathons.

In a file he keeps from people who send him letters, a grade-school student wrote, "Thank you!" in bright block letters in crayon after his visit. "My dad died of almost the same thing," she wrote. "He had heart problems. The bone around his heart was sticking out. He couldn't remember me or my family and he couldn't see very well and then on Oct. 16, 1997, everybody knew he is going to die that day and I told my mom I know he's not, I know it. The day before he died he toch my hand and squeezed my hand. It's like he knew he was dieing. Well after that my dad died and I didn't know what to say so I blamed God which I didn't mean to. It just came out because I was so mad and I wrote him a note saying, 'Dad, your eyes will always sparkle in everybody's heart' and 2 days later we had a funeral and I kissed him on the head and I said I love you dad with every part of my heart."

It was raining in Cincinnati and as we were driving, cars were whooshing by and constantly sending spray over the windshield. It was cool and damp—and Osterman was fed up with it. He and Carole would like to get out of Ohio and move to Florida, where he would spend less time with a wrench and more time attending running events and telling people his story. "I was never much of an outgoing person," he said. "After all of this stuff happened, I think I'm more involved with people. I feel better about myself. Before, I went to work, to the bar, and home, and I'd probably still be doing that. I know I wouldn't be in the shape that I am now. I probably would have been some butt-crack plumber."

DRIVEN

Osterman is in "better shape than 90 percent of the people who walk into a gym," said personal trainer Matt Hoffman. His business, Club Champions, caters to men and women who need extra help to get into shape. Osterman is different. He comes in, flips the switch on his favorite treadmill in the corner, and starts running. "He looks like this completely healthy forty-year-old guy and he's doing these crazy exercises," Hoffman said. "And then they find out that he is lot older than forty—that he had a heart transplant and he is a cancer survivor who runs marathons. They are just shocked. He's a great person to have around a gym."

When he started training for a marathon, Osterman would lift weights twice a week, concentrating on arms, shoulders, and back one day and legs the other day. He ran three or four days a week, gradually increasing his distance from 15 miles (24 km) a week to 60 or 70 miles (97 or 113 km). His weight would drop below 160 pounds (72 kg).

He turned to Hoffman because he was getting burned out. "He told me he felt as if he was just going through the motions," Hoffman said. He was hoping he could train smarter, increase strength and endurance, and lower his times. Hoffman moved him away from traditional lifting, such as biceps curls and the bench press, in favor of compound exercises that use more muscles and are done with little rest between sets.

One example: He starts with a squat and then moves immediately into an overhead press, all in a single motion. "An incredibly fatiguing exercise," Hoffman said. Osterman also does pull-ups and dips, squat and deadlifts. Strength-training sessions would take place on Tuesday and Thursday and last about 45 minutes. He would run three other days a week—often on a treadmill to avoid wear and tear on his joints. He starts with a preworkout nutritional shake with extra amino acids. After the workout, he uses a glutamine-based product to speed recovery and reduce muscle soreness.

"He is pushing it harder now," Hoffman said. "I think what happened is that there were times before, he wasn't sure if the weights would take away from the running. But what we found was working out hard for those two days was really helping with his running. He had a second chance with life, and every day he comes in here, you can see he's here to get into the best shape of his life."

Osterman's goal is to run 18 marathons—one for every year of the young woman whose heart is ticking inside of him. It's an admirable goal and has undeniable marketing appeal. But his last full marathon was the Flying Pig in 2002. His fastest was his first in Bermuda in 1998 when he was 43. He had been planning on the full marathon at the 2005 Flying Pig. But a month or so before the race he moved down to the half marathon. He had been having trouble getting in the requisite mileage because of demands at work and because he was spending more time with his mother, who had undergone hip-replacement surgery.

"Part of it for him is time restrictions," said Potapczyk, himself a survivor of a life-threatening accident in 2001 when he was 51. Potapczyk spent three days in a coma after a truck hit him while he was riding his bicycle. The collision lacerated his aorta and it took him nearly a year to recover. "I think after an accident you get leeway from employers and health care providers," he said. "Now he's got to work. And he does a physical job."

Surviving a Heart Transplant

When I first met Greg Osterman and his cardiologist, the 10-year survival rate for his 1992 class of heart transplant recipients was nearly 48 percent. The latest figures from 2007 show it's dropped to nearly 46 percent, according to the U.S. Health Resources and Services Administration.

Currently, the one-year survival rate is nearly 88 percent.

The five-year survival rate is just above 74 percent.

Recent heart transplant recipients have benefited from improvements in surgical techniques and drug therapies.

Osterman has bettered the odds because his transplanted heart was an unusually good match for his body. He assiduously followed his rehabilitation plan. He embraced exercise as a part of his recovery. And he was highly motivated—he wanted to get back to work to support his family.

The world's longest survivor of a heart transplant is believed to be Tony Huesman (born in 1957) of suburban Dayton, Ohio. He received his new heart at Stanford University in 1978. Huesman hasn't exercised as much in recent years because he has been hampered by various ailments. When he tells this to friends, "They tell me, 'what do you expect? you're in your 50s,'" he said.

In 2000, Osterman left plumbing and began working in building maintenance and currently works at Cincinnati Children's Hospital Medical Center. He moves through the halls pushing a cart, sometimes walking two to three miles a day fixing plumbing, heating, and air-conditioning problems. "Construction work was great, but I knew I couldn't keep this up for the rest of my life," he said. "I had to look after my health."

Vanden Eynden also moved over to hospital work. He said that stooping, bending, lifting, and working in all kinds of weather eventually catch up with most middle-aged plumbers. "I think he was feeling that he couldn't do it much longer—and do everything else he wanted," he said.

Osterman has never tried to push himself too hard while running. Because of that, he's never had a serious running injury. "I've never had a marathon where I felt really bad at the end—tired, but never really bad," he said.

Yet the months of preparation for a marathon were starting to become a chore. "The last marathon, it took a lot out of me," Osterman said. "I thought I would take a little rest and maybe regain a little bit of energy or muscle. It seemed like each one of them was taking a little more out of me. I thought if I cut back a little bit, I could get back into it a little bit further down the road."

But running has become a part of his life. Osterman continues to run in an occasional 5K race. He is working out three or four days a week—down a day each week from a few years ago. "Man, it's not getting any easier," he told me when we talked again in late 2008.

"I don't know what would take its place. It's a gift. If everything falls apart, if I go into rejection, I know that what I have done so far is the best that I could do. That's a good feeling for me to have."

8

Ironwoman

Laura Sophiea (born in 1955) plunged into Kailua Bay for the first leg of the 2007 Ironman World Championship in Hawaii and followed a friend through the chaos of arms and legs splashing through the water. Almost immediately two men—"big, rude, and mean," as Sophiea put it—swam over her. She panicked and began to tread water. Then she found a pair of quick feet and followed them until the three-quarter mark where she was kicked so hard in the nose and lips that she saw stars. She checked for blood and kept going. Sophiea always expects tumult in the swim of the Ironman and trains in the pool by swimming fast at the start of her workout and then backs off a bit in the middle before piling on strong intervals at the end to mimic the mad rush at the conclusion of the 2.4-mile (3.9 km) swim.

Next up, the bike. The 112-mile (180 km) ride is famous for its heat and winds, and in 2007 it was worse than usual. Aside from a 7-mile (11.2 km) stretch when the coastal breezes were at her back, Sophiea was buffeted by headwinds and crosswinds over the entire course. She saw one rider get hit by a car. Sometimes the wind was so strong over the lava fields that it pushed her bike at will. Usually cyclists share their annoyance as they pass each other. But on this day, they were quiet.

The marathon is what worried her the most. She had torn her hamstring some three months earlier. Sophiea was 52 years old and this was her 17th Ironman. She has fared remarkably well over the years while training for one of the toughest endurance events in the world. True, there was the time in 2000 when she competed in Ironman with a broken back. And in 1991, she wondered whether she would be suitably hydrated if she had to pull off the course and breast-feed her youngest daughter. But the run would be a test. She had spent hours getting massages to speed the healing of her leg. And she had practiced visualization to help her run pain free. She had backed off on her running from 35 miles (56 km) a week to 20 (32 km) in the final run-up to the race. She wondered whether the lower mileage would hurt her endurance or if all of the pounding would harm the hamstring.

It turned out it was the front of her legs, the quadriceps, that seemed tired as she transitioned into the run. She had already logged nearly an eight-hour day on the course. She was in first place in her age group. But the woman in second was only eight minutes behind. Mentally, miles 7 to 14 were the toughest in years—there was still so much ahead. As the miles droned on, so did the self-doubt. Why had she taken this on again?

She tried sipping a Coke, which helped her pick up the pace. In the final miles, she began feeling better and started to enjoy the race. As she neared the end, she could hear the music playing. I watched footage of Sophiea finishing the race on Ironman's Web site. Thousands of people lined Alii Drive in Kona and cheered as the athletes passed. The pace quickened as Ironman announcer Mike Reilly told the runners the clock was closing in on 11 hours.

The men and women around her were all younger. Most of the finishers seemed to ignore their fatigue and were bounding for joy as the end drew near. One man brought in his children for the final yards as athlete, son, and daughter held hands and crossed the finish line together.

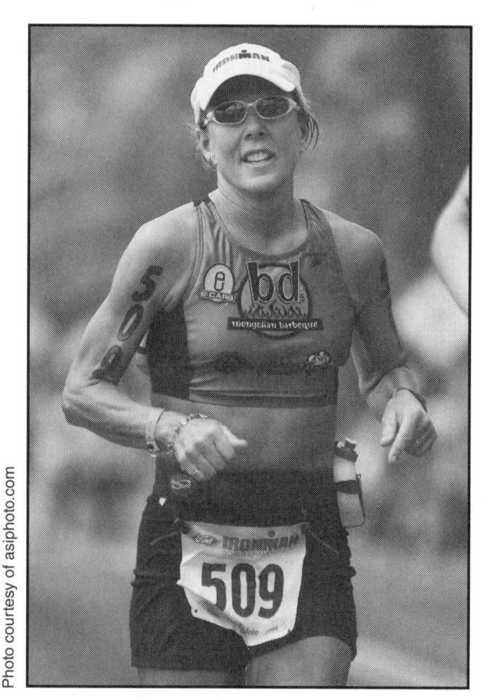

Photo courtesy of asiphoto.com

In her 50s, Laura Sophiea thinks she's in the best shape of her life.

"Laura Sophiea from Birmingham, Michigan," Reilly shouted over the loudspeaker as she rounded the corner and came into view. Sophiea was running strong, wearing a white sleeveless top and black running shorts.

"Way to go, Laura! Course record holder right here, 50 to 54! Laura Sophiea! Breaking 11 hours!"

Sophiea had won her age group in the Ironman again, coming in at 10:59:32, maintaining an 8-minute gap on her closest challenger. She pumped her arms triumphantly and smiled and waved to the crowd.

Then suddenly she veered sideways and started to fall. Two red-shirted attendants grabbed her and threw a towel over her shoulders. Then came a third, a fourth, and a fifth—all of them struggling to hold her up. In a moment, her joy turned to pain; the sparkle in her eyes grew as distant as a fallen prizefighter's.

Medical personnel rushed her into a tent, where two liters of saline dripped into the vein of an arm. An hour afterward, she vomited what little remained in her stomach.

For Sophiea, it was a typical Ironman finish. For all of her training and experience, each year she always bonks at the end, sapping every ounce of energy until it doesn't matter anymore. She told me her collapses at the Ironman do not bother her. She even viewed the extra liter of saline she received as a bonus—a gift—that helped her get back in the groove for her next race a month later in Clearwater, Florida.

Ordinarily, she would have flown back to Michigan a day after Ironman and sleepwalked her way through work for the rest of the week. But it had been a momentous year. She had taken a leave from her job as a librarian and media specialist at a middle school. Afterward, she stayed an extra two weeks in Kona to recuperate and resume training.

AGING SLOWLY

We met a few days after she returned home in late October to Birmingham, a Detroit suburb. Sophiea, at 5-foot-4 and 117 pounds (239 cm, 53 kg), could easily pass for a health-club-traipsing mom in her 30s. Training and a good diet had whittled her figure down from a size 10 to a size 2 over the past two decades. Her blond hair fell to her shoulders. Her skin was tan, her cheeks and nose pinkish from her stay in Hawaii.

Even though racing and working out have been an essential part of her life since turning 30, Sophiea considers herself to be in the best shape of her life. She recovered from the broken back—a transverse stress fracture of the sacrum, a bone at the base of the spine. And aside from the torn hamstring and the obligatory spills on the bike, she has rarely even pulled a muscle. She competes in about a dozen triathlons a year. In some, she finishes among the top women, regardless of age. She is most focused on Ironman in Kona—the Super Bowl of triathlons and the longest event she competes in. She won her age group for the first time in 2001 at the age of 46, making up a 25-minute deficit in the marathon. Her best Ironman time ever was 10:35:59 in 2005, at age 50. Her races in 2005, 2006, and 2007 have been among her fastest ever. In 2007, she finished ahead of all but two women in the next-youngest age bracket. The next year, she bonked again, but crossed the line in 10:38:46, nearly beating her best time ever.

Sophiea's ability to improve reflects a broader trend among some physically active women who are becoming stronger and exhibiting more endurance as they age. For many, their improvement comes because they have never done anything like this before. But in some cases, even veteran athletes are improving.

In the rarefied world of ultraendurance events, women are occasionally beating men outright. In 2002 and 2003, Pam Reed was the overall winner in the 135-mile (217 km) Badwater Ultramarathon that travels through Death Valley and eastern California. She was 42 at the time of her second win.

During a 10-year period, Ann Trason got faster running the 100-mile (161 km) Western States Endurance Run in the Sierra Nevada Mountains. She has set three age-group records in the race. Her time of 18:16:26 at age 41 was faster than her record at 29 of 18:33:02. In 1998, at the age of 37, she was the top finisher among all men and women.

Several factors explain this midlife renaissance. One is Title IX, which turned 35 years old in 2007. The law prohibits discrimination based on gender at schools that receive federal funds for educational programs. Athletic opportunities were still limited for Sophiea and her contemporaries during her college years, but the inexorable effect of the landmark law is that more women have begun to participate in sports than at any other time in history.

Old notions about aging have been thrown out the window, as well. "I firmly believe that we have underestimated as a culture, and maybe even in the field of exercise science, what older adults are capable of doing," said Miriam Nelson, director of the John Hancock Center for Physical Activity and Nutrition at Tufts University in an interview with the *Los Angeles Times* in 2007. "It's really important for people to realize that you should not underestimate what people can do based on age, gender, and chronic disease."

The effect of this culture change is that it's not uncommon for women, deep into adulthood, to find their inner athletes. And when they do, it can be an epiphany. "I had no athletic ability, no God-given talent," Sophiea told me. "But when I started getting better and winning races, it was empowering."

Reed said much the same thing: "When I won Badwater, women didn't just have to go after *their* race. Sometimes we could compete for everything and that's a very powerful feeling."

Women are also tapping into the latest advances in training and technique. Sophiea claims to train intuitively, but she has built up considerable know-how over the years. I would mention a study or an article that was related to endurance or aging, and she was familiar with it. She corrected me on a fact in a story we both read about marathon runner Alberto Salazar in the *New York Times* that recounted his famous duel with Dick Beardsley at the 1982 Boston Marathon. It wasn't four liters of saline he received intravenously, but six, she told me. I went back and checked. She was right. Given her experience with the IV bag, I should have known.

In her milieu, she is surrounded by men and women who are constantly trafficking in the arcana of equipment, nutritional products, and workout regimens they think will give them an edge. Sophiea owns five bikes, and she believes part of her recent success can be attributed to a new high-end Cervélo frame and the expert bike fitter who tweaked her seat post and handlebars. Her old bike was two centimeters bigger and not adjusted properly. "If you looked at me, I am more aerodynamic on the bike now," she said.

Staying Balanced

Jan Guenther (born in 1959) is a businesswoman, a triathlete, cross-country skier, mother, and wife. I first met her at the 2004 American Birkebeiner when she was 46. She and her husband own GearWest, a sporting goods store in suburban Minneapolis. For years she has been among the country's best cross-country skiers and triathletes in her age group.

"I love racing," she told me. "I'm trying to let go." She laughs. "I'm trying to let go, because my kids do not know how to play hockey and they live in Minnesota. And they don't know how to cross-country ski as well as they should. They need more time. They need more *me*. It's the same problem everyone faces."

Guenther's solution has been to find ways to simplify her life. She doesn't wear makeup and she keeps her hair cut short. In her view, a well-conditioned body is the best fashion statement. With so many demands on her time, she stopped using a training log and a heart-rate monitor. She trains as many as six days a week. But after turning 40, she found she needed more sleep and more time for her body to recover. She told me how she would meld exercise while playing with her two sons, who were then in grade school. A strength workout might be interspersed with the boys crawling over her. When she was outside with them, she would do quick hops and jog around the driveway. Tailored workouts have become less important than being outside with a group of like-minded women. "That's been really fun," she said. "You meet women who want to do good, who want to be strong, who are juggling a lot of things."

With time she had become mentally stronger, which allowed her to use her experience to decide when to push and when to hold back. She has cut down on her in-season running from five days and 50 miles a week to four days and 35 miles to save wear and tear on her legs. At the pool, she swims with a clock. Each set is calibrated so that she has a few seconds of rest before a new one starts. It is a workout designed to stress her body and thereby improve her ability to process oxygen and develop a higher tolerance to lactic acid, which builds up when the body goes into oxygen debt. Sophiea also has started using a heart-rate monitor again. In an all-day race like Ironman, she wants to make sure that her heart does not exceed 145 beats per minute; otherwise she is burning energy from glycogen, which can be sustained only for a short period.

When I told Sophiea that I fatigued quickly in the pool with a kickboard after only a few laps, she concluded that my ankles weren't flexible enough. She promptly sat down on the floor of the coffee shop where we were meeting, extended her legs straight out, and bent her feet forward until her toes touched the floor. I tried doing the same and fell short by several inches. This hyperflexibility allows Sophiea and others like her to turn their feet into big flippers to push them faster through the water.

Sophiea believes that her performances have improved since she has begun to eat mostly whole grains, vegetables, and low-fat protein, especially fish. She has eschewed red meat for years, and when she cooked it for her family, she wore plastic bags on her hands. Pasta and cheese pizza, made with refined white flour, had been mainstays of her diet. Cheese was her main source of protein, but she thought it was too fatty. "That's not a healthy diet," she said. She makes her own whole-wheat bread twice a week with a bread machine. She doesn't eat butter, which is high in saturated fat, but uses olive oil and canola oil. These days she is eating more fruits and vegetables such as spinach salads and fish as a source of protein in place of cheese. She has also become a devotee of recovery drinks and nutritional supplements. She said they have helped her recover faster in her 50s. She began using them even before her victories on the triathlon circuit helped her get an endorsement deal for free products from Hammer Nutrition.

Sophiea entered her first triathlon in 1985 when she was 29 years old. She decided to give it a try because one of her sisters and some of her friends were doing it. She was not exercising at the time. "Zero," she said. "I had been a cheerleader. I didn't know that I had a competitive bone in my body."

The first race was a half-mile swim (0.8 km), 12.4-mile bike ride (about 20 km), and 3.1-mile run (5 km). She borrowed her husband's bike, a Fuji, and practiced climbing a hill once. But she didn't know how to shift the gears and didn't even try during the race. She finished in the middle of the pack.

The next year, her husband bought her a Peugeot and she took up with a group of bicycle riders and learned the basics. "That changed everything," she said. "Once I started riding with men—faster men—that is when I started to get better."

One of the riders, George Tomey, now a principal in suburban Detroit, taught her to keep pedaling after cresting a hill. "Most people coast down the hill—never do that," Sophiea said. "You just keep going. That's how you drop people."

Tomey told me that they met on a 70-mile ride after Sophiea's first triathlon. The group they were riding with stopped for breakfast, but Tomey and Sophiea, who both had children, needed to get home. Tomey was a competitive cyclist and the best rider in the group. As they were riding back, she asked him if they could ride again.

"She's always sought out people she could sort of stay close to, but were faster, and that is why she rode with me," Tomey said. "She wanted a carrot. It didn't matter if she could catch me. She wanted it out there."

The two trained together for 10 years, often riding to the point of exhaustion. "You were pushing yourself, finding out where the edge is and getting as close to it as you can," he said of their training together. Tomey termed his own training then as "excessive" and eventually he stopped riding for six years because of a herniated disc that was partially aggravated by cycling and because the long hours on the road were taking away too much time from his family.

After her first triathlon, Sophiea had done well enough to qualify for the national triathlon championship at Hilton Head, South Carolina, in 1986. When she got home, she leafed through the list of competitors and looked for women from Detroit. She called Jan Jacobs. The two had never met but lived five minutes apart. Sophiea asked her whether she would like to start running and biking together. They have been cycling or running together ever since.

Jacobs is married with two sons and has competed in international age-group duathlons involving biking and running. She also has a master's degree in exercise physiology.

"Laura is definitely a person who knows what she wants and she doesn't much let anything stand in her way of getting that, which is a good thing," said Jacobs, who shares a birthday with Sophiea and is two years younger. "She is by far the most focused person I have ever met." This, coming from a woman who continued to work out well into a pregnancy, just as Sophiea did. At 43 and pregnant with her second son, "I ran and biked to the bitter end," Jacobs said.

Jacobs has been a personal trainer since 1989. "Sometimes when you first start with women, they feel guilty for taking time away from their family to exercise," she said. "And I tell them, 'Number one, you are going to be a better parent and a better spouse by doing this for yourself because you are going to feel better about yourself and have a better outlook.' You have to convince them of that."

Still, she could never be as devoted as Sophiea. "I can certainly relate to that sense of accomplishment, and how that keeps you coming back, because I have definitely experienced that," Jacobs said. She likened it to her training for the Boston Marathon before she was married. "The majority of my life had to revolve around it: my diet, my sleep, my social life. I was glad I did it. I had great races," she said. "But when it was over, I had to relax for a few months. I wanted to resume some things that I had put aside. I don't see Laura ever doing that. This is her constant lifestyle. And that's the difference. She never seems to need a change. It is her life. And I'm not taking anything away from her—she's a fabulous mother. She's a hard worker. When I met Laura, she had a master's degree. She was working on a second master's degree. She had a husband and two children and was working full time and training. And she was doing all of them excellently."

Sophiea's two oldest girls are in their 20s and swam in high school. The oldest was on the swim team at Michigan State University, where she was nominated as a Rhodes Scholar. Her daughter currently teaches high school in Ferndale, in suburban Detroit, and coached Sophiea's youngest daughter, a standout swimmer.

Sophiea separated from her husband in December 2005, moved to a rented house in Birmingham, and later divorced.

IRONMAN'S ROOTS

The first long-distance triathlon was held in 1978 in Hawaii. Its roots lie with a group of navy SEALs and endurance junkies in San Diego who had been getting together for swim–bike–run events for several years before that. Triathlons flowered in the 1980s, and Ironman's reputation as one of the most grueling events in the world was dramatized on national television in 1982 when Julie Moss crawled on her hands and knees to a second-place finish. Membership in USA Triathlon has risen steadily from 15,937 in 1993 to 100,674 in 2007, according to association figures. USA Triathlon estimates that up to 250,000 people try a multisport event every year in the United States.

Paula Larsen is a former national age-group triathlon champion who raced Kona in 2000 and finished fifth in her age group despite walking a portion of the marathon because of fatigue. In 2006, at 61, she was part of a four-woman cycling relay team in Race Across America, or RAAM, the virtually nonstop bike marathon from suburban San Diego to Atlantic City. She was part of an eight-person team in 2008.

Larsen believes the Ironman takes a special kind of person to thrive on its demands. "You need to do a lot of long-distance biking," she said. "You have to increase your run time. You have to get that swim time in. And you need to do bricks." Bricks are workouts when two of the disciplines of the triathlon, often a bike and run, are practiced back to back. "You bike 75 miles and then you run for 15 miles," Larsen said. "Do you know how many hours that is?"

"Laura is very, very focused on (the Ironman) and I guess, if you talked to me five years ago, you might have found me the same way. I've just relaxed a little on that. Sometimes I think that you just have to. At some point, maybe Laura will also. All it takes is one injury. At our age, one injury can really knock you out."

Sophiea estimated that at the peak of her training, in the three months leading up to the Ironman, she spends 18 to 20 hours a week working out. It helped that she had her summers off, but it was harder to stay on track in September when school started. When her three daughters were younger, it was even more difficult. It was not uncommon for Sophiea to read with her youngest daughter and go to bed by 9:00 and be up by 3:30 or 4:00 in the morning to get in her workouts. After school, she would leave the girls with their grandparents twice a week. On weekends, she would ride as much as 100 miles and be home before lunch.

When we met, Sophiea was getting ready for the World Triathlon Championship in Florida at a distance that is half of an Ironman—1.2-mile swim (about 2 km), 56-mile bike (90 km), and 13.1-mile run (21 km). She had left her house at 5:30 in the morning and was in the pool by 5:45 and swam 2 miles. She changed clothes and ran to the track for speed work. In the waning days of Daylight Savings Time, it was pitch dark in Michigan. She couldn't see her watch, but she estimated that she ran a mile in 7:15, two half miles in 3:20, and finally two quarter miles in 1:35. She ran a total of 7.5 miles before making a dentist's appointment at 8:00, then a doctor's appointment before meeting me at noon.

By 3:30, it was time to bike. Sophiea lives in a small ranch home on a tree-lined street in the throes of transition. For blocks, houses were dotted with "For Sale" signs. Detroit was hobbling through hard times, only to worsen with the ensuing recession, and yet old homes like the one Sophiea rented were being torn down and replaced with houses that were twice the size.

The sky was a brilliant blue and temperatures had soared to an unseasonable 65 degrees. Many of the oak trees on the block looked as if they were coated in honey; maples were lit by fire. Sophiea carried her blue-and-yellow Giant road bike out the front door as her friend Mary Ward straddled her own bike. The two of them would be heading out, passing the construction equipment and the twirling leaves to join a group of women for a 32-mile (51 km) ride from Birmingham. They did their best to avoid the snarl of traffic by combing through subdivisions north and west of town. As usual, Sophiea chose the route.

"Laura is a born leader," said Ward, who was 53 and a teacher in the same school district that Sophiea worked in. "She's not bossy. She's just the best rider among us and she always has a plan." Meaning that if it's a cycling day, Sophiea will be on the road. "I remember one day when I first started riding with her and it started to snow," Ward recalled. "Then it started snowing hard, and I thought, 'Oh, my gosh, she isn't going to go back.' Another time we biked in an ice storm and we came back and our helmets were all filled with ice. Our clothes were a sheet of ice."

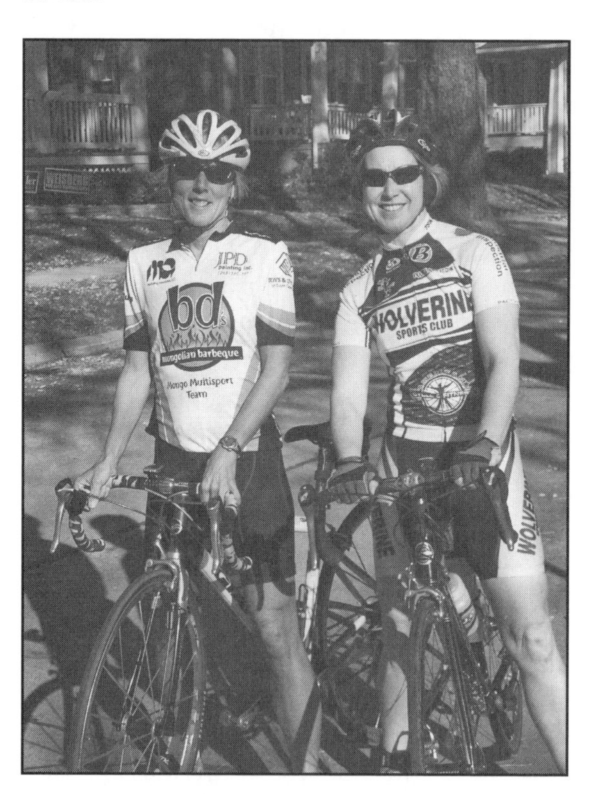

Laura Sophiea and Mary Ward prepare for an afternoon ride in suburban Detroit.

Tomey remembered riding with Sophiea when she was seven or eight months pregnant. "We were in some pretty ugly weather and there was that big stomach hanging between the handle bars," he said. "I thought it was a little shaky out there on the bike, but she wanted to get those miles in. That was just Laura."

Sophiea's push to excel is the key to her talent, he said. "She doesn't have a long femur bone like a great cyclist has," he said. "She is not gifted with great foot speed. I think she is gifted with great drive, which is typical of triathletes. They are not exceptional athletes in any one area; otherwise, they would just pursue that. But their drive and their discipline and their ability to tolerate the drudgery of training are greater than anyone else's."

In 1990, Sophiea entered a triathlon in Toledo, Ohio, in the middle of August. Her youngest daughter was born in January 1991. "Back then, they didn't want you to race," she recalled. "People said, 'You can't do this!' I said, 'Yes, I can!'"

A week after the baby was born (a 15-minute delivery), she was running and pushing a stroller. "Every workout she does has a purpose," said Jan Jacobs, who joined Sophiea and Ward for the afternoon bike ride. "She knows the amount of time she wants to spend and the intensity level she wants to be at for every workout she does. So when she walks out her door, she has a pretty specific idea of what she is going to do."

The ride took nearly two hours and it doubled as a time for everyone to catch up, since Sophiea hadn't seen her girlfriends since returning from Ironman. Afterward, they went out to dinner. Sophiea was home and in bed by 9:00.

Even though she was still feeling the effects of the time difference from Hawaii, she had managed three and a half hours of exercise that day, which is not unusual. "Obviously I am not a normal American," she said. "I don't watch television."

And I interjected, "You exercise!" I asked her if she was addicted to it all.

"Yes, I'm sure I am," she said. "I would certainly not like to say I was, but I am sure that I am. I like to do something every day. I just like the endorphin high that you get. I could smoke. I could drink. I could have other vices, I guess."

But scratch deeper and you find other factors that keep her going so hard. She said her biggest motivating factor was making sure she was up early so she could get her workout in. It seemed overly simplistic to me, but for Sophiea, her morning ritual gives structure to her life. It is so important that before we met she had written down the reasons why she was an athlete. First on the list was getting her kinetic day off on the right foot by exercising. In her mind, everybody else may be sleeping, but after having knocked off a swim, a bike, or a run, she was ahead of the game.

Her strict adherence to training then allows her to set goals. As she has gotten better, she has found that laying out her aspirations was how she got better. Each year, she wants to improve at Ironman. Much of her goal setting comes at improving her prowess on the bike, since cycling often produces the biggest gains in a triathlon. The payoff comes in places like Kona and other venues with a win or a high finish. It validates everything.

Ironwoman Tips From Laura Sophiea

Getting Going

Most women have false expectations. They start out too quickly with their exercise program, their bodies rebel in pain, and they quit. You should think about spending this much time on preparation:

Sprint triathlon (0.5-mile run, 12.4-mile bike, and 3.1-mile run)—three months

Olympic (0.93-mile swim, 24.8-mile bike, and 6.2-mile run)—four months

Ironman (2.4-mile swim, 112-mile bike, and 26.2 mile run)—nine months

Why Am I Doing This?

Ask yourself if you like the three sports. If you don't enjoy swimming or are afraid of the water, you might want to consider a duathlon, which involves biking and running.

Another option is to find three friends and enter your first triathlon as part of a relay. My second race was part of a team, and it was such a blast because it allowed me to concentrate on biking for one race.

The Most Important Thing to Remember

Make it enjoyable. The more fun you have, the more you will stick with your training plan, achieve your goals, meet interesting people along the way, feel good about yourself, look great, and (most important) accomplish your goal of completing a triathlon. This adventure will become a journey in your life that you will never forget.

Being Fit at 50

I learned that I needed more sleep. I used to get by on six hours of sleep or less. Now I try to get eight hours. It was harder when I was still teaching. When I was unable to get enough sleep, I tried to fit in naps on the weekend to catch up.

I found that recovery drinks do make a difference. I drink Recoverite from Hammer Nutrition, which has a combination of protein and carbohydrate. I pay very close attention to what I eat and drink after a hard workout. People underestimate the importance of proper nutrition and recovery products if they train every day. Nutrition and recovery products are actually the fourth part of a triathlon.

How Laura Runs at 52

I run fewer miles. I went from running five days to four days a week. I make sure that my easy days are really easy and hard days are really hard. Because I run shorter and longer triathlons, I do a mix of distance and speed work.

Speed. When I go to the track, I used to run mile and half-mile repeats at a 6:15 pace. Now I do them at a 6:45 pace.

Tempo. My 40-minute tempo run on Thursday includes a faster 22 minutes at my 10K pace, which for me is 7:05.

Endurance. I usually will run after a long bike ride on Saturday. I used to run 7 or 8 miles (about 11 or 13 km); now I will do 4 or 5 miles (about 6 or 8 km). We call that a brick. Then I run long on Sunday and try to set my pace close to an Ironman training pace of 8:15 per mile. A long run for me from May to August is up to 16 miles (25.7 km) and maybe one or two 20-mile runs (32 km) in September before Ironman in October.

Staying Healthy

Racing triathlons allows you to work three sports. Running is the hardest on your body. So now, after a hard running workout, I can ride a bike or swim the next day and let my body recover. I get massages every week in racing season and twice a month in the off-season. I take ice baths for recovery on my hard days (brrr!). The best thing I have done in the last three years is to develop my core body strength.

Sophiea's Web site is http://trimasterscoach.com.

Sophiea thinks her athletic accomplishments have helped to "show my girls that there is more to life than getting married and raising a family—that it is really important to find something that you love," she said.

Like many athletes, Sophiea uses exercise to help counteract what aging takes away. She doesn't wear it on her sleeve, but she is clearly proud of her youthful appearance. Looking and feeling healthy are important parts of many older athletes' self-image. And perhaps because it's such a critical part of their lives and they see people older than them who look so good, they find another justification to keep going. "I don't want to live an unhealthy life when I am old," she said. "I don't want my kids to see me like that."

Sophiea also finds herself emotionally suited to the kind of training that comes with triathlons, and she thinks that the variety has helped her avoid injuries. There are no endless hours in the pool or day upon day of only running. She ran only one marathon in her life and when she finished, she thought to herself, *That's it?* "I would never train for a marathon again," she said. "It's too one-dimensional—and there would be no reward in it," meaning she isn't fast enough to win her age group. She especially loves cycling and being outdoors. In the winter, she switches to a heavy mountain bike, which is safer on the roads and provides a harder workout.

Sophiea prefers not to work out alone, and by extension, her training partners and the triathlon subculture factor heavily into her social life. She reads voraciously but has few other outside interests. "I am not into interior decorating," she said. "I don't wear makeup. I don't care much about clothes."

In the fall of 2007, for the first time in 30 years, Sophiea did not return to school. It was a hard decision because she loved her job. Although balancing school and training and her family was challenging, she liked trying to keep it all together. The change has given her more flexibility to train and more time to sleep. When she was working, she was getting by on six and a half hours of sleep when she felt her body was starting to crave more. That fall, she was also making plans to start a business coaching women—especially middle-aged women—who want to train for triathlons.

Sophiea was also spending more time with Kevin Moats, an Atlanta developer and triathlete who is the same age as Sophiea and her male equal in the triathlon. Moats holds the record for the fastest time in the Ironman for men 50 to 54. At the 2007 world championships, he finished fourth in a division where the top few men are closely matched.

In the summer leading up to Ironman, the two were living a fairy-tale existence for those with a penchant for travel and exercise. In July, they spent three weeks cycling 800 miles (1,287 km) through the Alps and the Pyrenees and watching two stages of the Tour de France. They rode along the mountain stage of Alpe d'Huez, and on another mountain route, Col du Galibier, they pedaled amid the clouds and shared the road with grazing cattle.

Then it was on to Kona for a two-week Ironman training camp in August. Sophiea returned home to Michigan for a short time, then she and Moats flew back to Hawaii the month before the race to train, cycle the course, and acclimatize their bodies to the heat.

After Ironman, Sophiea returned to Michigan on several occasions to be with her daughter, once serving as a timer for a two-day swim meet. Sophiea and Moats planned to spend much of the winter together in Atlanta with a trip back to Hawaii and Wyoming for skiing.

"I met someone I really like," she told me. "We could have continued the relationship with me living in Michigan and him living in Atlanta, me continuing to work and seeing him on weekends. But if he has the ability to allow me to not work, it's worth trying it. I'm young enough, I'm healthy. Why not? I mean, I might as well try this stuff now. Why should I waste all of this time and wait until I am 65?"

Part III

The Long Haul

Speed and quickness are attributes of youth. But endurance sports favor older athletes. Over the long haul, patience and passion, grit and resolve are as important as the physical act itself. Eventually, an athlete can wear himself out. But often, it's the desire that burns out first. What motivates someone to run every day for decades? What keeps an athlete coming back after an endless string of injuries? Marathons are painful, so what drives a runner to keep doing them past the age of 85? There are many answers. But many athletes will tell you that they are addicted to it. And then they'll quickly add: "But it's a positive addiction."

9

Streakers

Some athletes burst on the scene with a sizzle and flash, and then like human fireworks, they burn out and are never seen again.

Others have a special kind of staying power. Aside from talent and genetic good fortune, their greatest attributes are their passion and perseverance. Some even go beyond traditional enthusiasms. They love what they are doing so much that they never stop.

In the world of running, this compulsion to keep going has manifested itself in a certain kind of person who runs every day. For some, the days turn into weeks, the weeks turn into months, the months turn into years, and improbably, the years sometimes turn into decades.

They are called streakers, and two runners, in particular, got my attention. In different ways, they are prototypes of the zeal and discipline required for being a streak runner.

Bob Ray (born in 1937) had the longest running streak in America before he stopped in 2005. He had run every day for 38 years and five days. In the process, he had worn out a marriage and 114 pairs of shoes. He was 68 when he stopped, and his once-feathery stride had disintegrated into a slow, bow-legged gait.

John Chandler (born in 1955) was 53 and still running smoothly. But there were nasty periods that nearly ended his string.

To an outsider, to run every day is at once strange and yet so natural. If we strap on a pedometer, many of us will find that we walk several miles a day. Running is merely an extension of this—just break into a trot and go. Little is required beyond a pair of shoes and a minimum of clothing.

But running *every day*—with its physical stress, the natural desire to go faster and get better, the demand on one's time—seems far more daunting.

It is one thing to run on a glorious day when the body is rested—indeed, coltish—and raring to go. But it's quite a different matter to try hobbling on an injured leg or to go out running when your body, your mind, your spouse, or a child is conspiring against you. It says a lot about why streaking is practiced by only a determined few.

America has a tradition of extreme running, said Richard Benyo, editor of *Marathon & Beyond*, a publication catering to long-distance running. He pointed to a six-day bicycle race at Madison Square Garden in 1909 and the "bunion derbies" of 1928 and 1929 when men ran from Los Angeles to New York City for prize money. Today, people run races of more than 100 miles. Ironman triathlons have been trumped by double Ironmans. "I think it's in people's nature to want to one-up what people have done before," Benyo said. "Man has always wanted to challenge himself, and when you look at our society in general, where so many people are not doing anything, they are just sedentary, this is sort of the other side of spectrum."

Streaking attracted little attention until George A. Hancock of Windber, Pennsylvania, himself a streaker for 24 years before he stopped, cobbled together the first comprehensive list in 1994 for the *Runner's Gazette*. In 2000, a group of runners formed the United States Running Streak Association Inc. and began keeping records. Today there are 189 members with active streaks and another 112 with retired streaks. (Please see appendix for the official USRSA streak lists.)

According to the rules of the association, a runner needs to run at least one continuous mile within each calendar day under one's own body power. They can run on a road, a track, or a treadmill. But runners can't do it with mechanical aid, canes, or crutches and they can't rely on the buoyancy of a swimming pool. Running fast, running for long distances, even winning a gold medal in the Olympics doesn't earn any extra credit. It's all about the streak.

The association has also devised a ranking system. It takes 5 years of running every day to emerge from the bottom rung of neophyte and move to proficient. From there, runners graduate to experienced (10 years) to well versed (15 years) to highly skilled (20 years) to dominators (25 years) to masters (30 years) and finally to grand masters (35 years).

Until Mark Covert of Lancaster, California, took over, Ray's streak was regarded as the second longest in the world behind former British Olympic marathoner Ron Hill, who has run every day since 1964. Covert's streak reached 40 years on July 23, 2008. It began in 1968 when he was 17. American troop levels in Vietnam had reached their peak and the Beatles' "Hey Jude" was the top-selling single. After 100 days, he realized he had a streak. Covert was blessed from the start. He was a gifted runner, loved running, and struggled little with the emotional and physical demands of his daily ritual. He still looks forward to running, but he admits his feet have been pounded flat by his obsession. After high school he ran his longest distance, 52 miles. He was a college All-American and finished seventh in the marathon in the 1972 Olympic Trials. Today, he is head track and cross-country coach at Antelope Valley College in Southern California. Other leading streakers are a writer, retiree, software developer, dietitian, dentist, attorney, and sales representative. They are all men in their 50s and 60s.

BOB RAY: RUNNING FOR THE RECORD

The first thing that intrigued me about Ray was that he didn't have a desk job for much of his streak. He was a letter carrier. During his streak, he had run an average of more than 7 miles a day (about 11 km), and before he retired, he walked another 6 miles (10 km) a day on his mail route. The walking might have been beneficial, since a common technique among long-distance runners today is to walk as a way to reduce atrophy and purge lactic acid from aching muscles.

Ray started running in high school in 1953 and continued to run regularly until the start of his streak on April 4, 1967, three days before his 30th birthday.

These were the days when running was a fringe sport. Frank Shorter would not win the gold medal in the marathon until the 1972 Olympics. Bill Rodgers and Grete Waitz had not yet burst on the scene. "People would look at me," he told me. "Cops would follow me home."

Ray's streak began with a 4-mile (6.4 km) run. He was wearing a pair of cutoffs and high-top tennis shoes and running with three women from work when one of them said she had run every day for two weeks. He wondered if he could do the same. Weeks turned into a month and a month turned into a year. By the end of the first year, he was running an average of 37 miles (almost 60 km) a week.

He has five hard-bound ledgers, two calendars, and one spiral notebook detailing his streak. Over the years he added more details. Since 1988, he has entered the month, the day's date, the time when he started, the temperature, a description of the weather, the number of miles run, the total number of miles in the streak, and the sum total number of days in the streak. He also kept a space for any sundry notes (a doctor's appointment, for example), and when I thumbed through it, I saw a note to buy

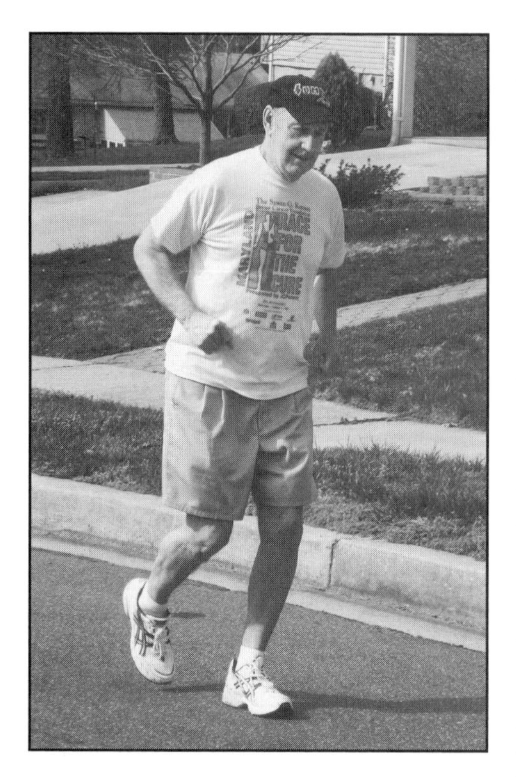

Bob Ray believes running has kept him centered.

cat food. Ray also kept count of his total "career" miles. He estimated he had run 22,000 miles (35,406 km) before the streak even started. Running was never a chore. One of the few times the streak almost ended was when he had to squeeze in a run at 10:30 at night after returning home from Alaska. He was flying back from a marathon.

During his streak, Ray ran 13,885 consecutive days and competed in more than 500 races, including 18 marathons. His mileage zoomed to 100 miles (161 km) a week for a time in his mid-40s when his marriage was crumbling. It was his way of coping. As the streak neared its end, he was running an average of 52 miles (83.7 km) a week, or nearly 7.5 miles a day. Ray retired from the postal service in December 1993, meaning he ran almost one-third of his streak in retirement.

He seems to have enjoyed keeping the records as much as he loved running. It involved order and discipline. It was a way of enumerating what was deeply woven into his life. "In a way, it's kept me on an even keel," he said. "It's helped me keep control of my life." Yet he could also find whimsy in it all. Ray has run races in a Spiderman costume and as an 18th-century admiral. In 1989 at a women's race he worked in, he wore a white tuxedo and parked his 1981 white Cadillac Coupe de Ville at the finish line. In 1990, he ran up 27 stories of an office building on Baltimore's harbor—barefoot—and came in second place.

In 1987, the year he turned 50 and hit his 50,000th mile (80,467 km) during the streak, Ray took a month off from work and drove cross-country for what he called his Tour of America. On July 4, he left Baltimore in a 1968 Chevy van that he had restored. His goal was to run in all 48 contiguous states.

With a mailman's eye for novel addresses, he picked burgs like Harmony, Minnesota; Hazel Green, Wisconsin; Mule Creek Junction, Wyoming; and Stone Mountain, Georgia. They were locales that not only sounded good, but they also pushed him toward his next state. At each stop, he would ask someone to sign his log after he had finished his run and hand them a T-shirt he had designed for the trip. On three occasions, he hit three states in a day. The most he ran in a single day was 19 miles when he covered Florida, Alabama, Mississippi, and Georgia. It snowed in Oregon and he labored through a steam bath in Arkansas. His favorite venue was a high school track in hot and windless St. George, Utah, at 2:00 a.m. He ran 10 miles in 74:56 on a red Tartan track. The craggy landscape felt like he was on the moon. The school's lights backlit arcs of water from the sprinkler as it went round and round on the grass infield as Ray ran around the track. His feet started getting wet and he finished the last mile barefoot. "It was beautiful," he said. "I thought I was in heaven." When he returned home on August 1, he had driven 9,232 miles (14, 857 km) and had run a total of 299 miles (481 km).

Ray Lorden, Bob Ray's running partner for 10 years, said that Bob's job was to pick the route and set the pace every day. "He's very goal oriented," said Lorden (born in 1954). "He plots everything out. I run because I love to run. I was the Forrest Gump. But Bob remembers times, dates, all of that stuff." On the day Cal Ripken Jr. of the Baltimore Orioles broke Lou Gehrig's streak of playing 2,131 consecutive games, the two of them ran exactly 21.31 miles.

It was all part of his running life. Much of his identity was rooted in it. His first wife resented it; running was one of the reasons he got divorced. "It was right on the edge—it was always waiting there as an issue," he said. In 1978, she joined him at a runner's meeting. "I remember her getting up and saying, 'How do you get a guy to stop running? It's me or his running,'" Ray said. "Well, I opened my big mouth and said, 'Where are my shoes?' I was as much at fault in the divorce as she was. I was stubborn enough to say, 'Look, I don't have to do everything you want me to do. This is something I do for myself.'"

He separated in 1984 and lived out of his van for two months as he struggled to make support payments for his wife and youngest child. The couple divorced in 1986. He never told his wife about the streak.

He met his second wife, Cindy, in 1992. He stays home while she goes to work as a legal secretary in downtown Baltimore. After they were married, he ratcheted down his running to his daily minimum of 4 miles (6.4 km) on weekends. Cindy has been more accepting of his running. It was a mistress she could live with. She did worry, however, about the wear and tear that all of the running had on his body and his vulnerability to inattentive drivers. "When he tells me that he had to jump out of the way of the car, that bothers me," she said.

They live in a brick single-story house on a hill in a subdivision northeast of Baltimore. The home is immaculate and he approaches housework with the same fastidiousness he brought to running. When I visited him, a neatly rolled-up American flag was leaning against a wall in the hallway. In the living room, a two-seat La-Z-Boy was stationed in front of the television where Ray watched his two favorite programs, *The Oprah Winfrey Show* and *Dr. Phil*. He has a stationary bike and an art studio in the basement where he paints idyllic landscapes on ceramic tiles. He's painted hundreds of them. After my visit, he sent me a lush painting inscribed "Maryland Memories" that depicts a brook and a series of small waterfalls that flow next to an old mill and a country road.

Runners are bound by honor to accurately report their streak tally. While we were sitting in the living room, I asked Ray if anyone had ever questioned whether he had really done it. "I've heard it before," Ray told me. "How do we know that you run every day? I ran places during my streak where no one ever saw me run. There is no way to tell."

He said he has invited doubters to watch him run or run with him. He never had any takers. He emphasized that he never sought the attention. The first articles written about him were in the mid-1980s, nearly 20 years into his streak. It wasn't until the mid-1990s that he started to become known outside of the running community.

"There is not a doubt in my mind he did it," said John J. Strumsky Jr., president of the U.S. Running Streak Association and a friend of Ray's. "Bob is as honest as the day is long."

Getting Organized

Strumsky was one of the founding members of the association with Ray, George Hancock, and Margaret O. Blackstock of Atlanta, who has been running every day since September 9, 1979 and has the second longest streak among women. In the beginning, the organization nearly dissolved over what constituted a streak. "We found that people were running around the kitchen table or down the block," Strumsky said. There were threats of lawsuits before members agreed on the 1-mile minimum. Today, most members run 3 to 10 miles a day, he said.

Another question streakers confront is this: Are they dedicated, or are they addicted to exercise? Most of the top runners I've read about agree that they are hooked on running, but they didn't see it as harmful.

"I think then you have to take the definition to the next level, and there can be two types of obsession or compulsion," Strumsky said. "There can be positive obsession, or there can be negative obsession. I think this is a positive obsession."

Strumsky has a running streak going back to May 23, 1983. In 2006, he ended his 15-year streak of running twice a day as a birthday present to his wife.

I visited Ray in April 2005 after he had decided to end his streak. He is bald on top with short cropped hair on the sides and a gray mustache. He looked younger than 68, but he had thickened around the middle compared to pictures I had seen of him a decade earlier. He told me that he didn't want to reach a point where he was running so many miles that he'd succumb to a streak-ending injury, or worse. He had kept running during two cases of walking pneumonia in 1977 and 1996. But aside from the usual assortment of a runner's aches and pains, he had been remarkably healthy. Yet after we were sitting for more than an hour, it was clear that running had exacted a toll on him. When he got out of the chair for a glass of water, he rose slowly and limped bowlegged into the kitchen.

Ray had been a "skimmer," a light-footed runner who saved a lot of wear and tear by not pounding the pavement. "In his early days," Strumsky said, "when he was in full stride in a race, the way I remembered him, he was just like a gazelle. He just glided over the ground like he hardly touched it."

Long-Term Effects of Running

Excessive running can cause injury, especially for runners with poor biomechanics. But running for decades does not have to be a prescription for such problems, according to researchers at Stanford University. Their longitudinal research in the August 2008 issue of the *American Journal of Preventive Medicine* found that X-rays of knees of 45 runners, compared with 53 nonrunners, showed no greater evidence of osteoarthritis. The subjects were evaluated between 1984 and 2002. Their mean age was 58.

"In 1984 when we first started this, there was a big concern that running may be good for the heart, but it's going to destroy the knees," said Dr. Eliza Chakravarty, an assistant professor of medicine at Stanford Medical School. "The data suggests that running didn't hurt the knees." It might be that the efficient stride of a long-term runner helps. Chakravarty also suggested that runners had strengthened muscles and ligaments and improved bone density compared to nonrunners. Also, the motion of running helped squeeze fluids through cartilage, keeping it lubricated and nourished. This is important because blood vessels don't feed the cartilage.

Ray told me his knees had become arthritic and would feel better after a few minutes into a run. "Ten years ago, the doctor told me I had the knees of a 27-year-old," he said. "But there has been deterioration since then."

On April 7, 2005, Ray kissed Cindy good-bye. A few minutes later we were jogging slowly on one of Ray's regular running routes. He hadn't slept well. He said he felt anxious about ending the streak. I could smell the Ben-Gay he had slathered on his knees. He wore a white hat, blue running shorts, a T-shirt from an old race, and a pair of his favorite Asics running shoes. Keys and dog tags with his name, phone number, and blood type jangled around his neck as he ran. In his left hand he wore a cutoff sock for wiping his forehead.

We ran down the hill from his home to the running track at the local high school. This was Ray's turf. He's probably run more miles here than anyone in the world. But school was in session, and he asked the PE teacher for permission to run on the track. He mentioned that it was the last day of his streak. The teacher nodded blankly. The girls were running 400 meters, but more than being winded, many of them seemed bored with it. How ironic: The girls were being introduced to running while an old man was putting in the final steps of a 38-year streak. They thought of it as drudgery; running had defined Ray's life.

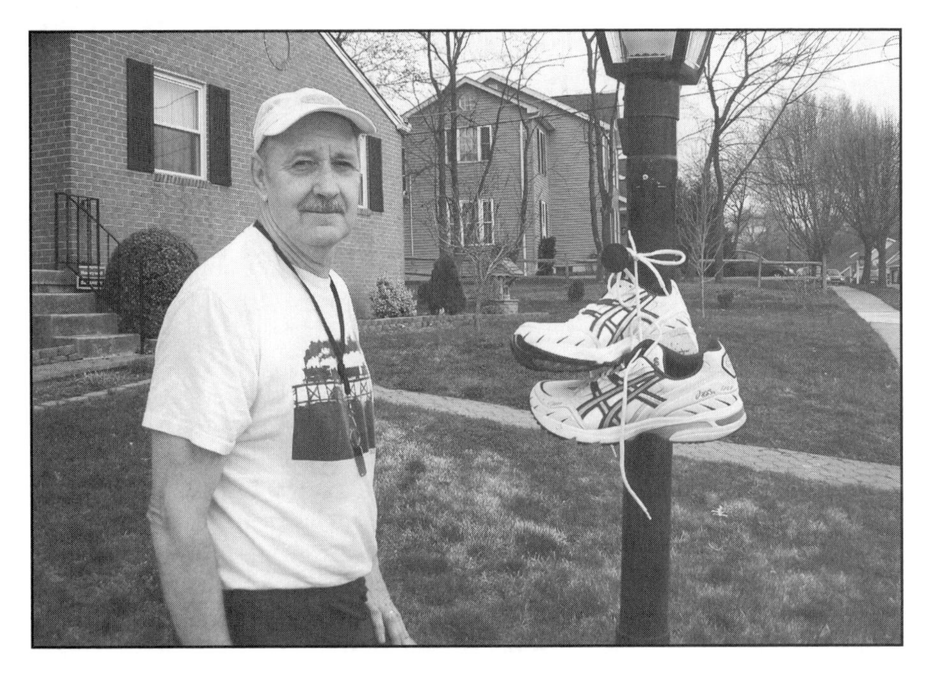

Bob Ray ceremoniously hangs up his running shoes at the end of his streak.

He talked almost nonstop, often repeating stories he told me the day before. We ran a leisurely pace, 10- or 11-minute miles, and we were soon heading home. With a few blocks to go, I told him to go ahead. I slowed to a trot and watched his pace quicken as he ambled up the hill. For weeks, he had calibrated the length of his runs. The last day of the streak would cover 4 miles (6.4 km). He had drawn a line on the street with green chalk in front of his house and when he crossed it, Ray had run exactly 100,000 miles (160,934 km). I shook his hand. Then he took off his shoes, tied the laces together, and hung them on his lamppost in the yard. He was finished.

Postscript: Life After Running

I called Ray later in the summer. He was still running occasionally, "but I've cut way back," he told me. The Tour de France was in progress and he watched the race each day as he pedaled on his stationary bike. When he noticed Lance Armstrong and other riders picking up their cadence, he did too. "It's fun to imagine you are pedaling with them," he said. "I try to see if I can catch Lance."

Ray quit running altogether on December 18, 2005. It was exactly 52 years after he started. In 2008, he underwent total knee replacement surgery for both knees. Toward the end, running was "like hitting your toes with a hammer," he said. "It feels so good when you stop." Since he stopped, his knees have felt better.

Cindy said that her husband no longer had the pressure of keeping up the streak. "I think that he is more relaxed now," she said.

Ray described his streak as a lifestyle that became an obsession that became a lifestyle. "One follows the other," he said. "It was something I had to do. It was like being a trained rat. I still miss it in a way."

JOHN CHANDLER: I'M A RUNNER

On the morning of December 27, 2003, John Chandler was working on a puzzle with his daughter when he heard an incredible sound go off in his left ear.

He turned and said to his wife, "Whoa! What was that?" But the words came out in a jumble. He tried to say he was fine, but Mary called 9-1-1. The ambulance arrived in two minutes and took him down Lake Drive, a street that runs along Lake Michigan and is a popular spot for runners on Milwaukee's north shore. At the time, his streak had been going for more than 22 years.

"I remember seeing the other runners going down Lake Drive," he told me. "See," he recalled telling himself. "That's why I like to run first thing in the morning, because if you have a stroke later in the day, you've got the run taken care of."

Chandler, who was 48, was having a transient ischemic attack—a mini-stroke, a warning that a full stroke could eventually follow. He didn't know it at the time. He was given an electrocardiogram and a doctor concluded that he was fine. Later that day he went for a 5-mile (8 km) run and kept the streak intact.

In July, it happened again at the bathroom sink. He dropped his toothbrush, twice, and felt a sharp feeling like an electrical current in his right cheek and then a sensation like a shot of Novocain. He went ahead with his plans to join a group for a 12-mile (19 km) run that day.

A running friend, a doctor, advised him to get further tests. He learned that he had a small hole in his heart that had not closed when he was born. In most babies, the hole closes after they are delivered. If it remains open, it can allow a blood clot to flow to the brain, which can lead to motor control and speech problems. He had these options: He could take a drug to reduce clotting, undergo a surgical procedure to close the hole, or do nothing. He opted for the medication, but as he considered surgery, he reasoned that he might be able to go for a run at 1:00 a.m. the day of the procedure and run again at the end of the next day.

"I didn't think it was the end of the streak," he said. "The streak runner is optimistic."

Chandler's streak began on August 9, 1981. By the end of 2008, it was the 55th-longest streak in the country. To keep it alive, in 1992, a sympathetic doctor changed the time for surgery to remove a kidney stone so he could squeeze in a run. In 2004, a bout of flu had left him badly dehydrated and so dizzy he couldn't stand up. One of his running buddies, another doctor, drove him to a hospital and directed staff to put a bag of saline into his arm. A few hours later he was able to get his run in.

And then there was the night when he ran through his neighborhood as Mary was having contractions. He would circle back every half-mile to see if the bedroom light was on—a sign that it was time to go to the hospital.

Chandler broke his left ankle in 2004, of course, while running, turning it on the curb to avoid a couple who had been walking their dog. He had pulled ankle ligaments plenty of times, but this time it was different. "As soon as I did it, I started swearing that it was over," he said. "I really did it this time."

The next day, an orthopedic surgeon he knew from college examined him. The doctor asked whether he still had the streak going. Chandler said it was.

Could he try running on it?

He could try. It could cause more damage, but maybe not.

Chandler wanted to try running on it. His final hurdle, however, "wasn't getting to the track," he said. "It was getting past Mary." When he got home, he told her that doctors thought it was broken, *but they weren't sure*, because one view of the X-ray had not been conclusive. Chandler said she called him stupid, and I can imagine her rolling eyes and her muttering words like *stubborn* and *men*.

Later, she described her husband to me as "your basic type-A personality . . . and you pick your battles and this is what he wanted to do."

He strapped on a walking cast as tightly as he could and at 8:00 he went to the local high school track. It was a windy, rainy night in December in Wisconsin.

He wanted to run eight laps—2 miles, or 3.2 km—his personal minimum for a run. But after eight steps, he knew he'd never get that far. He settled on trying to finish four laps—a mile and the minimum required for streakers—by putting almost all of his weight on his right leg. He finished in 12 minutes. The next day he ran a mile again and lowered it by a minute and then by another minute the next day. For the first few weeks, he would drag himself out of the bed in the morning, unable to put any weight on his foot. He ran a single mile for 44 straight days before he started dialing up the mileage again. By comparison, ordinarily he was running an average of just over 6 miles a day, and more in the summer, to get ready for a marathon in the fall.

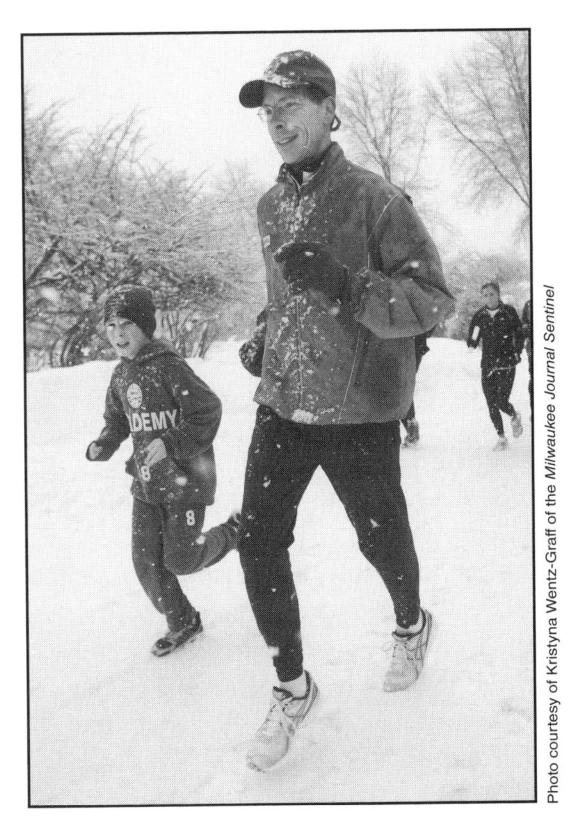

Photo courtesy of Kristyna Wentz-Graff of the *Milwaukee Journal Sentinel*

John Chandler with son Jack on December 24, 2008—10,800 days into his streak.

Origins of a Streak

Chandler played tennis and ran cross-country at Lawrence College in Appleton, Wisconsin. The streak began while he was working on an MBA at the University of Wisconsin–Madison. He checked his running diary and realized he had run every day for 10 days. "Then it turned into two weeks, and then two months, and then two years," he recalled.

In the early days, he squeezed in his runs at 11:00 at night. "I was still struggling with it a bit," he said. But now it is very rare for him to run at the end of the day. "It would hang over me—knowing that I still had to do it," he said. "Somehow I treat it as a given that I will slot it into some part of my day."

I didn't know that he had a running streak when I first met him. He lived only a few blocks away and we served together on the board of a day care that was housed in a neighborhood United Methodist Church. (The Chandlers' two children are now in grade school.) He was, in my view, a regular guy who wore nice suits and worked downtown. He had a financial background and had obvious leadership skills. We made him president of the board.

Over time I learned about what he called his "silly little streak," "this intriguing little toy," or "something that has become part of my persona."

I remember at a Cub Scout meeting in the December 2005 he looked ghostly pale—a shadow of the energetic dad I had come to know. He was weak and his back had been killing him. As a gym full of boys darted around us, he rasped, "I don't know how much longer I can keep this up." What he meant by this, he later told me, was he didn't think he could keep running and be sick for three or four more *months*. If it dragged out that long, he'd have to quit. I learned later that he was sick for 50 days, missed four days of work, and lost 10 pounds on his 5-foot-10, 145-pound frame (178 cm, 66 kg).

Chandler has had various running ailments over the years, but none that he considers debilitating repetitive-stress injuries, and nothing like the troubles that sidelined Bob Ray. He runs about a minute-a-mile slower than he did when he was 40. The slower time is a result of age, he said, not running every day. If he wanted to improve his times, he would run harder—not take days off.

"I love to run—most days," he said. "There are some days that I will come back and Mary will dutifully say, 'How was your run?' And I'll say, 'I didn't feel like a runner today.'"

Chandler can tell you about his first race—in fifth grade. His best marathon was a 2:37:37 when he was 29. (By comparison, a runner who sought to compete in the 2008 Olympic trials needed a time of at least 2:22.) At the age of 51, in 2006, he ran Milwaukee's Lakefront Marathon in 3:10:00—a 7:15-mile pace—and placed fourth in his age group for men 50 to 54.

He runs at 5:30 a.m., at lunchtime, or Sunday mornings with a group of other runners. An average run takes about an hour. He likes the reflective periods that it affords. But Chandler is a social animal, and often when I see him, he has been motoring at a quick clip with other runners.

In late 2008, it dawned on Chandler that Christmas Eve would mark 10,000 consecutive days in his streak. On the morning of December 24, as snow fell in thick, wet flakes, I joined Chandler and 20 other runners for a jog through the neighborhood to commemorate the achievement. Fittingly, the distance would be 10,000 meters (6.2 miles). The weather in December had been brutal. A few days prior to our run, with the forecast calling for the wind chill to plunge to more than 20 degrees below zero, Chandler had stayed up late, leaving the house at 12:05 a.m., in order to get in a 7-mile run before the temperature dropped. On the Christmas Eve run, road crews were having trouble staying ahead of the snow, so it was like jogging on a soft, sandy beach. However, our group seemed largely oblivious to the conditions. Afterward, we all stood in the middle of the street in front of Chandler's house drinking coffee from large urns and wolfing down donuts from the back of his minivan. He had handed out laminated maps at the beginning of the run, and on the flipside, he provided some statistical context to the streak. Chandler had run about 65,000 miles. He had worn out more than 100 pairs of running shoes. He had run in more than 20 marathons. His streak, still going strong, had lasted for 27 years. By now it had lasted more than half of his life.

In addition to his job as a financial planner, he volunteers as an assistant coach of a girls' high school track and cross-country team. He runs with the girls once a week and is on hand for all their meets. His eyes glistened when he described for me in exacting detail how one of his runners nipped another girl by less than a half-second to win the 3,200 meters at the state championship in 2006. (She was on hand two years later for the Christmas Eve run.) When he was in the ambulance after his first transient ischemic attack, his pulse registered 45 beats per minute, and a paramedic explained to another paramedic that the low number was because Chandler was a jogger.

"I'm *a runner,*" he mumbled in protest.

Scott Jenkins, a friend of Chandler's and a former All-American in track and cross-country at Wisconsin, said that Chandler is one of the most disciplined runners he has ever met. They ran together in Madison and in Milwaukee when he was vice president of stadium operations for the Milwaukee Brewers. He now works for the Seattle Mariners.

"I have been a runner all of my life, and I can't imagine running an entire year without taking a day off," Jenkins said. "Just to do it every day, think of the personal toll—there are work issues and family issues. It takes a special kind of person to get up every day and make it happen."

On an average day, Chandler doesn't feel any different than he did 10 years ago. "In a way it's kept me young," he said.

And what would happen if it all ended? "Would I survive? Absolutely," he said. "Would I be the same person? Yeah. But there would be a certain something missing."

Adapted, by permission, from J. Bergquist, 2006, "It's a long run: Bay area man hasn't missed a daily run in 25 years—and is passionate as ever," *Milwaukee Journal Sentinel*, August 8, 2006.

10

Swimming Against the Tide

When Gail Roper (born in 1929) started swimming again in the early 1970s, she was getting in on the early days of the masters movement and the awakening fitness boom. Middle-aged housewives were trying out flip turns, sharpening their forehands, and entering road races. Sports let them reclaim a bit of their youth. It made them feel better. It was a way of transforming their lives—if only for a weekend at a time.

Roper was an Olympian and a national champion in her youth. She has set 292 national and 93 world age-group records over the past three decades. She specializes in shorter events, but she's highly versatile, and in recent years she's won everything from a 50-yard sprint and a 1,650-yard freestyle in the pool to longer events in open water.

But for all of her mastery, she has struggled with the countervailing forces of injury, indifference, and even outright hostility. Roper now believes she trained too hard in her 50s and paid the price with a debilitating neck ailment that nearly put her in a wheelchair. She never found a coach who fully appreciated her abilities. She has been divorced twice—marriage and swimming never seemed to mix. Her second husband was so opposed to her traipsing off to meets and practices that he would flush her swimsuits down the toilet.

We met the first time at the U.S. Masters Short Course Championships in Santa Clara, California, in 2001. She was 71. "You got another frustrated swimmer here," she said. "Second chance in masters swimming."

We were sitting in the shade as the sun glistened on the water at the George F. Haines International Swim Center. The scent of sunblock and chlorine filled the air. Wave after wave of swimmers dived into the water, their arms oscillating wildly as hoots and whistles from the crowd commingled with the sound of thrashing water and an old-time jazz band.

It is the storied pool complex where Donna de Varona, Don Schollander, and Mark Spitz once trained and competed. Swimming is littered with the bodies of burned-out teens who tired of the interminable workouts that are as much a part of competitive swimming as the water. Schollander left his own family in Oregon to attend high school in Santa Clara during the 1960s so he could swim under the legendary George Haines. But in 1968, after swimming in two Olympics, he was so disillusioned by the long hours of training that he retired. He was 22 years old. He was convinced that swimmers and their coaches would have to find a better way to train in fewer hours. "Your life was so dull," he wrote in his 1971 memoir, "so mechanical, so impoverished emotionally and intellectually, that you begin to feel like a robot."

There's no doubt that many of the swimmers at the masters meet in Santa Clara felt that way at one time in their lives. Many middle-aged swimmers I've met have told me they got tired of the pool and needed to get away from it for a while. Then they come back. Men and women in their mid-30s to 50s make up the largest proportion of masters swimmers. Around the age of 40, many hear the ticking of their biological clocks, and now that their kids are getting older, they feel they can spend an hour or two in the pool for three, four, or five days a week.

At Santa Clara, parents would be racing one minute and holding the hand of a child the next. In a sport where buoyancy helps, it was not uncommon for amazingly fast competitors to spill out of their Speedos. Inevitably, the age-group athlete is in a war of attrition; as swimmers move up in age brackets, their numbers diminish. By the time they hit 70, even in the big national and international meets, a relatively hardy few remain.

"Gail is one of the swimmers who are redefining what it means to grow old and be an athlete," said Bill Volckening, editor of *USMS Swimmer* magazine, a publication of United States Masters Swimming. "We really don't know what swimmers at these ages are capable of," he said. "Gail is one of those who have kind of led the way."

"She's certainly been an inspiration to me," Peggy Sanborn told me in 2006 while I was visiting a retirement center in Santa Barbara, California, where she taught an exercise class in the center's pool.

Sanborn (born in 1927) is a sculpted backstroke specialist who competes in the same age group as Roper. She routinely finishes in the top 10 in national meets. But because of a spinal injury in her 50s, she spent months sleeping in traction and didn't start swimming competitively until she was 64.

"I'm not in Gail's class," she said. "I've talked to her about technique because she knows so much. To me, it's much more natural for her. I really think that swimmers who trained at a young age are just naturally more competitive."

THE EARLY YEARS

Roper began swimming in high school in the late 1940s. In gym class, girls could swim only one length of the pool before they had to get out and rest. The boys, of course, were doing laps, swimming them fast, and piling up the yardage.

Young Gail Peters had heard that the captain of the boys' team had swum a mile—72 lengths of the pool—so one day when the teacher left, she tried swimming a mile. Nearly 50 lengths into it, the teacher returned. She was incredulous and demanded that Gail stop immediately. Didn't she know that swimming so hard was bad for her heart—that her ovaries could burst?

"Ladies didn't swim fast," Roper recalled. "And they didn't swim very far. It was considered unladylike."

Turning 80

Gail Roper turned 80 in 2009, and early into the year she broke six world records. "Turning 80 was a motivating factor," she said. "It hurts when I swim, but it's worth it." Arthritis has reduced her mobility. Her oxygen uptake has also weakened in recent years, so she needs to take more breaths between strokes, which slows her down. Roper and the small cadre of competitive swimmers who are 80 and older are pioneers. Roper wishes there was better information on pool workouts for someone her age. "How does one train at 80?" she asked. "How much is overtraining—if you hurt all the time?" Roper doesn't think the answer lies in technology. At the 2008 Olympic Trials in Omaha, Nebraska, she and other former Olympians tried out one of Speedo's new LZR Racer suits, which Michael Phelps wore when he won eight gold medals in Beijing. It took her a half-hour to get into the suit. It was so tight around the chest, she thought she might be having a heart attack. Once in the water, the suit felt more buoyant—but it didn't make her swim any faster.

But she kept at it, with Lincolnesque rigor, swimming against the current of the Delaware River near her home in Trenton, New Jersey. She watched the better swimmers and read all she could find on training and technique. She became a New Jersey state champion at 19. She moved to Washington, D.C., to work in drafting and swam for the Walter Reed Hospital team. By 1952, at the age of 22, she became a national champion.

Roper's slight physique belied her prowess in the water. A *Life* magazine writer described her as "scrawny" in a 1952 story on the Amateur Athletic Union championships in Daytona Beach, Florida. "She looked anything but athletic" in her pink-rimmed glasses with rhinestones. "But in the water, she looked wonderful, and as champion after champion suffered heartbreaking losses, Miss Peters became the star of the meet."

Roper won the Olympic Trials in the breaststroke and was swimming's nominee for the Sullivan Award as the nation's top amateur athlete in 1952. That year in the Helsinki Olympics, she got a glimpse of sports on the world stage where men such as distance runner Emil Zátopek of Czechoslovakia were the center of attention and women figured in as bit players. Gail and the other female swimmers didn't stay in the Olympic Village; they were relegated to quarters at a local hospital. Her own Olympic hopes died quickly when she pulled a ligament in her ankle and never made it past the quarterfinals.

The next year she beat the Olympic goal medalist Eva Szekely of Hungary to gain the number-one ranking in the world. She was again a nominee for the Sullivan Award and was looking to the Olympics in Melbourne in 1956. But the rules were changed and the breaststroke and butterfly were separated into two different strokes and Roper struggled with the new butterfly that used the dolphin kick. "I was swimming the old butterfly with a breaststroke kick and they sort of cut me in half," she told me. "I would have to learn to swim all over again, plus the coaches that told me I was being greedy to try to make two Olympic teams."

She moved to Japan, worked for U.S. Army intelligence copying maps, coached swimmers, and then retired from swimming at age 26. She married, divorced, and married again. She raised seven children and for years the closest she got to swimming was dragging her kids out of bed in the morning to coach them at the local pool.

Roper has a "huge competitive spirit and workout ethic," said friend and fellow swimmer Grace Altus of Santa Barbara. "She didn't get an Olympic medal, and she has been making up for it ever since."

"Different things drive different people," observed Phillip Whitten, former chief media officer of *Swimming World* magazine and the current executive director of the College Swimming Coaches Association of

America. "In Gail's case, by chance, she was denied an Olympic gold medal. I think there is something inside of her that wants to prove that she really is the best."

"Things were different in those days," Roper said when I visited her home in Healdsburg in Sonoma County north of San Francisco in the summer of 2006. "You were supposed to be a housewife. But I'm not a housewife—I'm a goal setter."

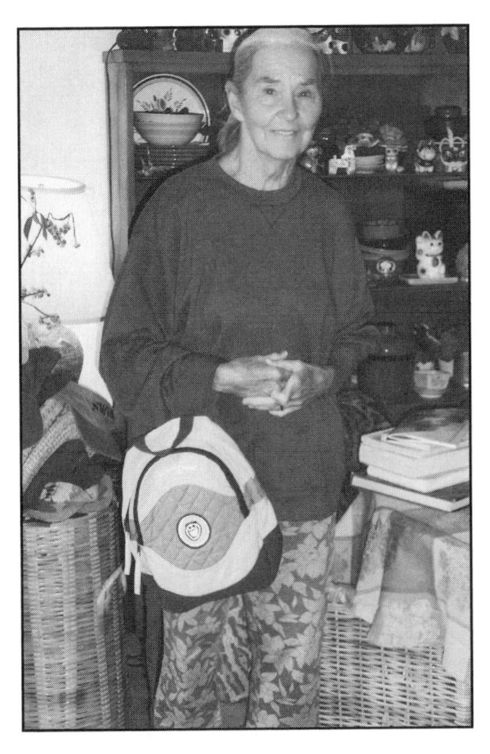
Gail Roper at home in 2006.

Roper was taking out the trash when I drove up to her rented bungalow in a subdivision that caters to older adults. She was then 77. She wore pink capri pants and a gray sweatshirt. She had let her hair grow since I had last seen her and it fell in a long, white ponytail to her shoulders. She had the same spark in her eyes I remembered from our first meeting more than five years earlier.

Her home is filled with books on nature, history, travel, art, and of course swimming. She has been to Africa twice and India three times. The influence is evidenced by zebra-print pillows and faux tiger and leopard skins draped over furniture. She uses a spare bedroom for her office, which is crammed with her computer and work files, figurines from her travels, and photographs of her children and grandchildren. On the wall is a faded photo from the 1952 Olympics.

Outside the window of her office is a bird feeder in her small leafy yard. Roper is a birder and had more than 600 birds on her life list.

"I have another life," she told me. Roper works full time conducting fishing surveys for the Pacific States Marine Fisheries Commission. She didn't start a professional career until she was 50. After Roper's second divorce, she moved to Hawaii and lived on welfare for four years. And then at the urging of a local women's organization, she took an entrance examination for college and got the second-highest score. She started attending a community college and eventually moved back to California and graduated from Sonoma State University. Her ex-husband raised the kids while she finished school.

"It was heartbreaking, but it's how I got my education," she said. "My life depended on my getting a degree. How else was I going to support myself? I was away from my children. It was one of those pills I had to take."

She supervises a field staff of eight along the northern California coast. She started at the agency before graduating from Sonoma State at 54 with a bachelor's degree in environmental studies. In her office, a pile of reports was ready to be processed. She wanted to get at them, but she knew I had made the drive from Silicon Valley two hours to the south. More important, one of her daughters, Samantha from New York, was making an impromptu visit and we'd be meeting her and another daughter for lunch.

Roper can be standoffish or she can wrap you in a hug. I've had trouble getting her to respond to phone calls or e-mails, and other times she will talk about herself with brutal honesty.

She carries a bit of a chip of her shoulder. I think it's what helped make her so good at swimming and drove her to start a professional career when so many others her age were starting to look toward retirement. She is proud to have gone to the Olympics but quick to say it was an injury that kept her from top form. Coaches either were misogynists or favored others. As an older swimmer, she has never been able to find one who treated her as a serious athlete. Marriage and raising kids, she will tell you, were a drag on her swimming career.

"It was an awful situation for me. I am kind of a romanticist—I like to do things," she said. "I like to see things. And I was a prisoner in the house."

It can be easy to forget the prevailing attitudes of the times—and even earlier when Roper was trying to become an athlete again. Over her husband's objections, she entered the first Senior Olympics in Los Angeles in 1970. She was 40 years old and couldn't make it across the pool swimming the butterfly. She won some races, but an old rival beat her in one event. Roper remembers the woman jumped up and down and yelled, "I beat her! I beat her! I beat her!"

"All of a sudden, something revived me—this competitive spirit," said Roper, her face turning serious. "That was the last time she was ever going to do that."

Swimming rekindled dormant emotions. The pool had made her strong. It gave her an identity. She had been a champion.

"I remembered who I was," she said. "I remembered who I was before I got married and trapped in the house. I used to go places. I used to go to swimming meets. I used to meet interesting people. I felt good about myself because I was getting exercise."

A CHAMPION AGAIN

She divorced in 1975 and soon became unstoppable in the pool. From 1974 to 1978 while competing in the 45-to-49 age group, she held virtually every short- and long-course record for most of those years. Roper was inducted into the International Swimming Hall of Fame in 1997.

From Phil Whitten, I heard about Roper's appearance on the *Phil Donahue Show* in 1984 and a documentary that featured Roper and a running Catholic nun in 1987.

Roper sent me a DVD of both. The women in the audience of the TV show clearly admired Roper and the other women who were on the program, including tennis star Billy Jean King. But I also sensed the confusion and frustration in their lives when it came to exercise. One woman said her husband didn't like it that she had taken up running. She wondered if her jogging would cause bladder problems. Another wanted to know whether she would bulk up if she lifted weights. Another runner stood up and said she had been told to stop because it would make her breasts sag.

My chance to see Roper swim at the peak of her middle-age prowess was in the 1987 Lynn Mueller documentary *Silver into Gold*, which was nominated for an Academy Award. The film featured Roper and Sister Marion Irvine, a Dominican nun and distance runner who was the oldest woman, at 54, to qualify for the Olympic Marathon Trials in 1984.

Roper had then what I saw decades later: a hunger to improve within the context of age. She was swimming long and hard, but she wasn't merely piling up yardage. She had adopted many of the training regimens used by the best swimmers of the day. On land she used a contraption with hand pulleys that mimicked arm motion in the water. She practiced visualization, pretending to stroke through the water before a race. She wore hand paddles for more resistance. In one scene, mist hovered over the pool as Roper, then 55, undulated like a dolphin. In the 1952 story in *Life* magazine, the writer said flip turns were often "too tiring for most women." But three decades later, Roper was executing them as smoothly as a dancer doing a pirouette.

When you observe the sheer competence of someone like Roper or Sister Marion, it's tempting to think it all comes so easy. But peel away the layers and you begin to see the schizophrenic mind-set of an older athlete: One moment they think they can do anything; the next they are acutely aware of their diminished abilities.

"I never think of my age as a swimmer," Roper said in the documentary. "I'm a swimmer. It's the same feeling I had when I was young and when

I was 40." Yet Roper got to the soul of the aging athlete in another comment. "I really want to go faster all of the time," she said. "I believe I can. But sometimes my body doesn't respond. What's happened to me? Why have I slowed down? It's aging. You just have to accept that."

Roper had been swimming up a storm. In the 50-to-54 age group, she set 16 world records and 54 national records. In the 55-to-59 age group, she set 12 world records and 38 national records. In hindsight, she believes she trained too hard during her 50s. Using techniques such as hypoxic training—not taking a breath over 5 to 10 strokes—made her go faster. But she thinks it unduly taxed her body.

By 57, her times began to slide. She thought more training would turn things around, but it didn't. She was diagnosed with spinal stenosis, a narrowing of the spinal cord that pinches nerves, causing pain—sometimes extreme pain—through the lower extremities.

"One doctor said, 'Don't take this spinosis lightly; I'm talking wheelchairs,'" Roper said. He urged her to see a psychiatrist and get used to living the life of an invalid.

At 60, she was forced to stop swimming and took a second job coaching the University of San Francisco Masters, a team that trained in a 50-meter pool on campus. The woman who never found a coach she liked was a no-nonsense leader with a waiting list for swimmers who wanted to get in.

"I didn't take fitness people," she said. "Everyone was there for fitness, but they had to compete."

A Roper rule is that everyone had to swim in at least one meet a year. When they got there, they usually found that Roper had signed them up for more events than they thought they were going to swim. Practice on Saturdays wasn't mandatory, "but they had to show up regularly," she told me. She took attendance.

"It was a love–hate relationship," recalled Duke Dahlin, who trained with Roper when he was in his 40s. "You'd love to hate her," he said. "But you were swimming so good, you never could. Every year that Gail was the coach, I got better."

In 2003, at 55, Dahlin swam the English Channel on his second attempt. He believes Roper laid the foundation for his 14-hour, 37-minute crossing.

Dahlin was pushed harder than at any other time in his life. He remembered a series of punishing intervals—10-100s on 1:15, meaning a swimmer had to swim 100 yards 10 times. Each new 100 started at 1 minute and 15 seconds, so the faster the finish, the more time for rest. But if swimmers pushed too hard, they risked bonking.

Training Under Coach Roper

Duke Dahlin keeps meticulous records of his workouts, including his days under Roper. The 1.5-hour workouts in the cryptography of swimming provide insight into the sophistication of Roper's training methods.

Wednesday Night, February 2, 1994

Warm-up (400 free, 400 kick, 200 free + 200 free/pull)

8 × 50 kick/free on 55 sec

4 × 75 free on 1:00

4 × 50 free on 45 sec

3 × (5 × 100 free on 1:20 + 1 × 500 free/pull)

8 × (25 kick/drill on 40 sec + 25 fast swim on 20 sec)

100 Cool-down

Here is some interpretation of the above: All of the distances are in yards. *Kick* means using the legs only with a kickboard. *Pull* means using only arms, not kicking the legs. Roper usually allowed about one 1 minute of rest between sets, so the body never fully recovers.

"I was 43 years old and I never thought that I could have done that," he said. "It was never boring. She kept mixing it up and challenging us." Not only were the workouts tailored to build endurance, but the emphasis on interval training helped build strength and speed as well.

AN INDEPENDENT SOUL

Coaching was a second job. Practice for the 200-member USF Masters was early in the morning or after work. Roper ran both sessions. She was living close to her job with the Pacific States Marine Fisheries Commission in Menlo Park. But it was 20 miles from the pool. A one-way commute in heavy traffic could take an hour or more. Roper would get home after 9:00 p.m. and had to be back at the pool in San Francisco by 5:30 the next morning.

So for five years, she lived out of her Toyota pickup truck, sleeping in the camper in the back around the campus, across the street from the university's health center and on Parker Avenue near Geary Boulevard. She rented a storage locker in Menlo Park so that she could stash her belongings and change clothes. She showered at USF and kept some of her personal effects at her USF and work offices.

"I didn't really need a house," she said. "I was saving all of this money. I couldn't swim anymore, so I thought I'd travel."

She had received $15,000 from a local bank after it had lost her Olympic participation medal that managers of the bank had showcased in the lobby during the 1984 Summer Olympics in Los Angeles. With the windfall and her accrued savings, Roper began taking her children, individually, to exotic destinations or places they wanted to see.

Roper would occasionally tell her swimmers how people would try to break into her car while she was sleeping, Dahlin told me. "At first I couldn't believe it," Dahlin said. "But she was working so hard, it became a fact of life."

Even after she stopped coaching and got a house, she continued to sleep out of her truck on trips. Friends told me about meeting Roper at swim meets, and to save money she would spend the night in the back of her truck.

"She is very much an independent soul," Grace Altus told me. Roper was a houseguest of Altus's in Santa Barbara in recent years. "She prefers to sleep in her car," she said. "But out of courtesy, she slept in the house."

John Morales, who was coached by Roper in his youth and has remained friends with her, recalled a time near Redding in Northern California when she swam a one-mile and two-mile race and slept in her truck that night. Roper was about 72 at the time. Morales and a group of other swimmers saw her at a rest stop on the way back home. It was hot and she was sitting in her car, a little groggy.

"We asked if we could help," Morales recalled. "She said, no, she was OK and was just going to rest for a bit. I swam one of the two events. She swam both. I stayed in a hotel and she stayed in her truck. That's one tough lady."

At USF, the hours of standing on the pool deck seemed to worsen her stenosis. She was having trouble walking and was thinking about using a walker. "I told myself, 'I can't do this,'" she said. "I've got to get back in the water."

She started competing again at 65 and soon began dominating her age group. When she came back, she didn't train as hard. Swimming had exacerbated her spinal problems, but now she believes her comeback helped to improve her condition. "The key is to train sensibly, to train smart," she said. "You get old—you are an aging athlete. Things happen. Cars are made out of metal. But even they wear out."

We drove into downtown Healdsburg. It was almost noon on a Friday and the town square was buzzing with weekend activity. Roper carried a light-blue backpack emblazoned with a "Life Is Good" logo.

She got a pacemaker in 2003. She also has neurological troubles. Some nights she wakes up and her hands are numb, probably related to the spinal stenosis. She has dialed back the intensity of her workouts even more. A few years ago, she was swimming four days a week. Now she was swimming three days a week and had cut back her yardage by about 25 percent to a little more than 1 mile per workout.

I asked her what her greatest strength was as a swimmer. She paused and after several seconds she said, "I have good genes. I have good flexibility. I float well. I have had to work hard on my technique. People say, 'Oh, you are just a natural swimmer,' and I say 'No, I'm not.' I've trained many years to work on my technique. The natural ability is that I float well. I have good flexibility in my shoulders and ankles. Other than that, I have to work on everything."

The night before, she had been watching a Webcast of American swimmer Michael Phelps in the 200-meter freestyle at the national championships. "I have worked for years to get my elbows up and last night I said, 'What's he doing? He had his elbows up.' That is kind of what I have been doing. I am still working on my technique."

But this neurological disorder was weighing her down. Her training had suffered and I thought it dulled her competitive fire. The 2006 FINA World Masters Championships were going on in Palo Alto, two hours away, but Roper was staying home.

Sometimes she'll scratch from the event when she hears a swimmer tell her that the two of them are going to have a good race. "I don't like to race people," she told me. "I hate it when people say that. I don't want to be put in that position where I have to be worried about somebody. I do my own thing in my own lane, and if I get a certain time and it's a record, wonderful."

I've seen this view of competition in other masters athletes. Some say they compete only against themselves, and then they hit a new age group and things change. Roper told me she was looking ahead. She would be 80 soon. By aging up, there will be new records, new challenges. "I've got to fix my neck," she said. "I've got to avoid stress. I'm just doing maintenance (workouts). I've got to make it to 80. I'll do therapy—whatever it takes."

In the park, two of Roper's grandchildren (Cameron, 9, and Sophia, 3) come running toward us. Roper gives them both a big hug. Daughter Sarah Quider, then 39, is a winemaker and lives a few miles away with her husband, Kevin. Roper often babysits for the couple. Samantha, the daughter who is visiting from New York, was 40.

We walked to a restaurant, and after we settled in, Sarah and Samantha told me about their childhood when their mom coached them. Samantha said her mother was the first to get up in the morning. Mimicking her mother's voice, she said, "Does anyone want to get up with me and go to practice this morning?" Everyone giggled.

To this day, Samantha associates hot dogs and hamburgers with the grilled food she ate at swim meets. "My mom is a very complex person," she said. "I think I understand her more now that I have to work and balance other things in my life."

Roper then poked fun at Samantha for getting so excited at the 2000 Olympic Swimming Trials they attended together. Samantha vowed to

Diving In

To become a better swimmer, you need to train harder and make improvements in your stroke. Joining a masters swim team is a good way to ensure you will accomplish both. In many communities, there is usually only a single age-group swim group, so shopping around for coaches may not be an option. Many masters I've talked to have emphasized that it's better to practice with other age-group swimmers than to join a youth team. Good masters coaches want to get the best from their swimmers. But they recognize that older swimmers must balance training with other demands in their lives and need more rest between heavy workouts.

Melinda Mann, who has broken world age-group records in the 50-to-54 age group, trained with her children's swim team after a decade of being away from the pool. She slipped easily into the regimen because she had competed at Michigan State University. Then Mann switched to working out with a woman who was 18 years younger. The two of them pushed each other to swim harder. Mann also began to pay more attention to her stroke than she had in college. Both factors helped her break the world records, she said.

If you are on your own, check out United States Masters Swimming at www.usms.org. The organization offers considerable information on technique in the form of articles (including *USMS Swimmer* magazine), a message board, and video rentals.

Bill Volckening, editor of *USMS Swimmer,* said that interval training is a key to improving. The idea is to swim harder than your usual pace, perhaps trying to swim a specific distance at a prescribed time. Then rest. Volckening suggests avoiding increasing distance by more than 10 percent per week.

join masters and start training for the next national masters meet. They shook on it, but Samantha eventually stopped training.

"Oh, Mom!" she said. "I hear this story all of the time."

Sarah recalled the blissful moments lying in her swimsuit under the sun. She can still smell the wet pavement beneath her. But it was hard to get up some mornings and go to the pool. "I remember hiding underneath my bed because I didn't want to swim," she said. "I wish I would have kept up with it."

"Why didn't you keep up with it?" Kevin asked.

She shot him an annoyed look.

"Other things came up, *like kids*," she said. Sarah had also gone back to school and finished a degree in viticulture and enology (the science of wine and winemaking) from the University of California, Davis three years earlier.

Roper sipped a glass of wine. The tapas rolled in like clockwork, each more delectable than the last. Sophia cuddled up next to grandma and was singing softly. Roper looked at the couple and said quietly, "She'll get back to it one of these days."

11

Racing Across America

Randy Van Zee's practice ride was coming to an end. He had started at 6:00 a.m. the day before, and now, 26 hours later, he was winding down the final miles of his nonstop ride across Iowa. He had not slept since he got on his bike, and he showed no signs of fatigue from 498 miles (959 km) of constant pedaling.

In fact, the ride had gone well: No flat tires. Traffic hadn't been bad. He had a bout of nausea in the middle of the night, but a cup of chicken soup and a warm Coke fixed him up. The trip in July 2005 had been a tune-up for the next year's Race Across America (RAAM). He needed a few training sessions like this one—constant cycling, no sleep, the white noise of the road—to help condition his mind as much as his body for the transcontinental race.

He was hoping for a better outcome. RAAM had battered him badly the first time he rode across the United States in 2004. His kidneys shut down. His neck muscles were so shot that he was forced to wear a brace to hold his head up. And the seemingly simple act of gripping his handlebars had reduced the strength of his handshake, even months later, to that of a young boy's.

As he rode through the night, he passed thousands of slumbering bicycle riders who were on a bike ride of their own: the 2005 Register's Annual Great Bicycle Ride Across Iowa, commonly referred to as RAGBRAI, a weeklong caravan of cycling and revelry. While they slept, he traced the riders' next-day route, flying through burgs like Spillville, Jackson Junction, and St. Olaf. The moon danced across they sky as he moved down one country road to the next until, finally, the fields slowly brightened and the sun burned its way into another summer day. As cars occasionally sped around him, his legs turned with seemingly little effort. He was eating up asphalt at a good clip, passing beaten-up barns, yarded-up Holsteins, and soybeans that looked like so many rows of neatly planted shrubbery. The edge of northeastern Iowa, perched above the Mississippi River, affords a sweeping vista of the valley below, and Van Zee was moving over it at a clip of 20 miles an hour (32 km per hour). Then, with his bike light flashing, he dropped into a steep, 400-foot plunge, coasting downhill at 40 miles an hour. It had been mostly smooth riding, but now newly caulked sections of the road were like little speed bumps, making his wheels go kurplunk! kurplunk! kurplunk! until finally the road flattened, he turned a bend, and then another, and glided into the sleepy river town of Guttenberg, where RAGBRAI riders were expected to arrive the next day.

I had been trying to shake the cobwebs out of my head as I raced to meet Van Zee. He was riding with a support crew, Gayla Vaandrager and Steve Moos, who had been motoring behind him in a light-silver Chevy minivan ever since they left Le Mars, in northwestern Iowa. Vaandrager had called me the night before and said that Van Zee was making better time than they had expected. He would be arriving in Guttenberg in the morning, not at noon as they had thought. This meant I would have to leave home in Milwaukee that night. It was a beautiful summer evening. I had been riding my bike through the neighborhood with my son and I still had work to finish before I left town. By midnight, I was on the road and speeding toward Iowa. My day had been a blur of activity—in a way, much like Van Zee's. But as he pedaled, I sat in front of a computer screen. When he and his crew got lost in the night, I was driving on cruise control. He had the music of crickets and cicadas. I listened to fulminating pundits on the radio. Finally, the long day and the longer night were all too much for me and I pulled over for a few hours of sleep. All the while, Van Zee was riding along at a clip that most men his age couldn't maintain for 15 minutes.

In the final miles, we met up—a dazed writer sticking his hand out the window, a lone cyclist quickly churning past me and offering a perfunctory how-do. I followed the flashing lights of the minivan into town and we pulled over on to River Park Drive. There was a park across the street, and beyond, the Mississippi flowed by us. He climbed off his bike, one of his favorites, a blue Trek 2500, which is built out of aluminum and was outfitted with a set of aerobars to reduce wind resistance. He was wearing a light-orange jacket, a darker orange shirt, and black Lycra tights. He

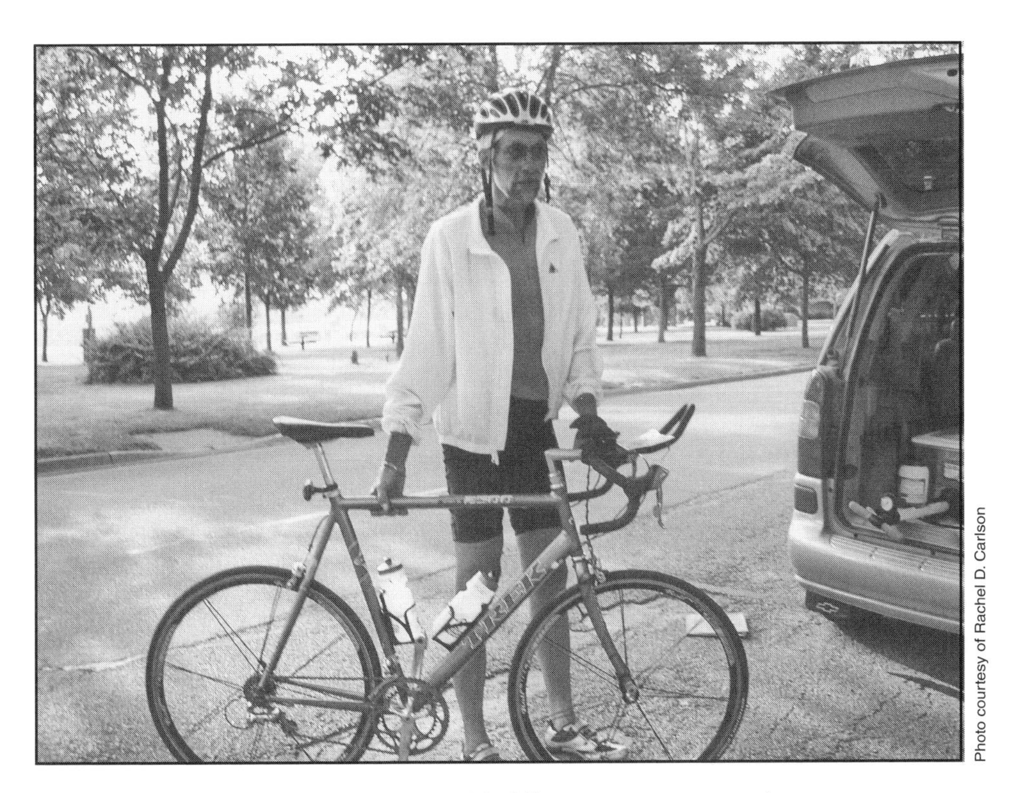

Photo courtesy of Rachel D. Carlson

Randy Van Zee in 2005 after riding his bike nonstop across Iowa.

didn't immediately stand out as one of the most aerobically conditioned middle-aged men in America. He was 53 years old (born in 1951). His face was tan and weather-beaten. He had a thick, gray beard and tinted John Lennon–style glasses. His legs were long, sleek, and shaved as smooth as a model's. He was also decidedly thin—a bean pole at 6-foot-3 and 175 pounds (190.5 cm, 79 kg). Later, he told me he was on "full feed." For breakfast alone, he knocked down three or four boxes of cereal a week, mixing the yin of Alpha-Bits and Sugar Smacks with the yang of Shredded Wheat and Raisin Bran to stoke an engine that bicycled eight hours a day, every day. Team Van Zee took over. A folding chair was quickly pulled out of the back of the van, and he sat down without saying a word. Steve Moos pulled out a large ice chest and handed him a can of cold soda. Vaandrager asked him how he was feeling, though she knew it had been a good ride—a sign that his training for RAAM in 2006 was going well. He had experimented with a new all-liquid diet, but he was still feeling hungry. His support team seemed anxious to head back home, but Van Zee wanted to go out for breakfast, and afterward stop at a hotel and sleep for a few hours.

AN EPIC RACE

RAAM has been described as one of the most brutal endurance races in the world. In 1993, *Outside* magazine examined other long-distance races that take place under harsh conditions—the multisport Raid Gauloises, the Iditarod sled dog race, and Vendee Globe, the 23,700-mile (38,141 km) solo sailing race. The magazine concluded that the cross-country RAAM was the toughest.

The race began in 1982 when four cyclists started at the Santa Monica Pier and didn't stop pedaling until they reached the Empire State Building nine days and 3,000 miles later. By comparison, the Tour de France, one of the most demanding events in the world, lasts for three weeks and covers 2,200 (3,541 km) miles. After leaving the California coast, RAAM riders soon find themselves battling the heat of the Mojave Desert, then the Rockies, the interminable Great Plains, more mountains in the Appalachians, and then a final scramble to the seaboard.

Amazingly fit cyclists in the prime of their lives have been reduced to lying down, puking their guts out, and bawling like babies. Many push themselves so hard during 22 hours of riding each day that they tap into IVs of saline as if they were filling up on gas. Most don't sleep for the first 36 hours, and many start hallucinating. In New Mexico, Van Zee said that boulders suddenly turned into wild hogs that would dart in and out of the road. "I can remember seeing their fangs, their teeth," he said. "They shined in the moonlight. They weren't dangerous or menacing. They just kind of came up there to see what was going on and then slipped back down. They were just playing a little game with me."

RAAM is at the apex of an ever-expanding universe of ultramarathon events. The 26.2-mile (42 km) marathon has become commonplace and eclipsed by even longer and more grueling runs, such as the Badwater, a 135-mile (217 km) race in California from Death Valley to Mount Whitney. The Ironman—with its 2.4-mile (3.8 km) swim, 112-mile (180 km) bike ride, and marathon length—has been outdistanced by the three-day Ultraman, which is more than twice as long. In 2007, 18 of Ultraman's 27 contestants were 40 or older.

The irony of competing in a solo bicycle race across the United States is that it takes a support crew to do it. Van Zee relied on six people during the first crossing, and his team believed it could do better the second time around. "Preparing for an ultramarathon ride is more like preparing for an expedition to the top of Mount Everest than a bike race," Michael Shermer, a former race director of RAAM, advised potential candidates on the race's Web site. (In fact, several RAAM riders have climbed Mount Everest, and one, Andrew Lapkass, who had his toes amputated after one ascent, says that RAAM is tougher than Everest.) There must be "meticulous attention to every detail," Shermer said.

"You have lots of points of failure," observed Lon Haldeman, the winner of the first two RAAMs, in 1982 and 1983, and a former official of the race. "If it isn't the lack of sleep, it's the saddle sores or your nutrition. RAAM is about controlling your problems."

Van Zee's team members learned a lot the first time around in 2004—everything from stretching his beat-up quads and streamlining logistical details to managing their rider's time. "Last time it was eat, shower, and sleep," Vaandrager said. "Now I think we will go eat, sleep, and maybe shower." At night, RAAM riders depend on the lights of a support vehicle to guide them down the road. It wasn't until Van Zee and his crew started that they learned that one team member had a sleep disorder and would fall asleep while driving as their man pedaled into the night. "He would fall way behind and Randy would have to wave him up and then he would fall back again and then he would have to wave him up again," Vaandrager said. She is a third-grade teacher at a Christian elementary school and an emergency medical technician for the ambulance department in Rock Valley, in western Iowa, which is near Sheldon, where Van Zee lives. She's known Van Zee and his wife, Denise, ever since she taught

Race Across America

Slovenian Jure Robic has won the race four times—in 2004, 2005, 2007, and 2008. He was 43 years old when he won the race in 2008.

New entrants must qualify to enter RAAM. One way is to compete in a 24-hour race. Men aged 50 to 59 would have to cover 400 miles (643.7 km), or an average of 16.66 miles per hour, to qualify. Sleeping or stopping to rest would require a faster average time.

In addition to the solo category, there are two-, four-, and eight-person teams. Organizers say it usually requires a crew of 8 to 12 people and two to four vehicles to get a rider or a team across the country. The cost of entrance fees and organizing a support team is about $20,000.

RAAM bills itself as the world's toughest bike race. The distance and nonstop nature of the event award cyclists who can endure pain for days on end with little sleep. Ultraendurance events might attract athletes who feel less discomfort, and it could be because of the way their brains are wired. At Wake Forest University Baptist Medical Center, brain scans of subjects whose skin surfaces were exposed to heat of 120 degrees Fahrenheit showed less activity in the pain center of the brain than others.

their children in school. Moos, a farmhand, was supposed to shoot video. But he jumped in to handle more duties when it became clear that others weren't up to the task. "They didn't look at it as a race," Moos said dismissively. Van Zee nodded and his eyes hardened. "They just didn't get it," he said. "This is RAAM—you know. You have to get me across. Forget about your agenda for these two weeks."

This was tough talk for Van Zee. For a race like RAAM, self-absorption is as much a part of the armor as a finely tuned body. Van Zee is warm, gracious, self-effacing—certainly inspiring—and in his own way, charismatic. Aside from his constant training, his annoyance about a few members of his old crew—almost a year after the race—exposed the intensity that boils inside of him.

FOR PRACTICE, A RIDE ACROSS IOWA

The citizens of Guttenberg had been preparing for the riders of RAGBRAI arriving the next day. The park along the Mississippi was immaculate. Lawns were trimmed. Flags were flying everywhere. Signs had also been posted along the street, welcoming the riders and pointing them to the river. For those who have been pedaling, partying, and sleeping on the ground for seven days, their final act is to ceremoniously dip their front tires into the Mississippi.

"Are you done with the ride?" a woman asked Van Zee and his crew.

"Yeah," Van Zee yells back. "We took off yesterday morning. We did it in one day."

The woman was confused. "Oh, you just did one day?"

Van Zee smiled. "We did it *all* in one day."

She smiled. Big joke. "Oh, sure you did," she said and walked on.

The same thing happened later at breakfast as Van Zee chewed on a pile of pancakes the size of dinner plates. The waitress asked if he was part of RAGBRAI. He repeated that he had just finished riding nonstop across Iowa.

"OK," she said blankly, moving to the next table.

He laughed and made a motion with the palm of his hand over the top of his head: The act of getting on a bicycle and riding for almost 500 miles goes right over most people. In Randy Van Zee's world, there are two kinds of people: those who understand his obsession with long-distance bicycling and those who can't fathom going so far for so long.

Van Zee began jogging in 1978 when he gave up tobacco as a birthday gift to his wife. He smoked cigarettes and a pipe and chewed tobacco. "I was addicted to smoking and I hated being controlled by that stupid weed," he said. "I couldn't make a phone call or have a conversation without lighting up. It bugged the crap out of me. I really wanted to quit." His weight zoomed to 270 pounds (122 kg). In the beginning, he could jog only a couple of blocks before he was winded. His crotch got raw from the fat on his legs rubbing together.

Van Zee admits there are addictive traits in his personality. When he quit smoking, he traded nicotine for a runner's high. He seldom took a day off and began logging the mileage of a world-class marathoner: 10 miles in the morning and another 10 miles after work. His first race was a 10-miler. He ran in dozens more, including eight marathons. His best marathon time, at age 36, was just under three hours.

But the pounding took a toll. His knees began to ache and he got sharp pains in his upper hamstrings. In 1989, he turned to speed walking and raced in several national speed-walk competitions. The hamstring troubles resurfaced, so he began a regimen of cycling and speed walking. By 1990, at 38, he switched to cycling altogether.

Van Zee has been flipped off by rednecks, had beer bottles and firecrackers thrown at him, and occasionally been chased by dogs. When we talked by phone one day, he told me that he had hit a dog, a rat terrier, the night before while riding near his home. It happened at a house he had passed many times before without incident. But this time the terrier decided to go after him, and it rolled under his tires and headed home with its tail between its legs.

He rarely rides with others. His turf in northwestern Iowa is one of the windiest places in the country. To the west are rollers along the Rock and Big Sioux rivers, which are tributaries of the Missouri River. In all other directions he is surrounded by row crops and flat and open roads.

The hours on the bike are a time for reflection or simply for living in the moment. "I love solitude," said Van Zee, a vocational rehabilitation specialist for the State of Iowa. "I value that—it's a personal value that I have. I am constantly dealing with people—either face to face or on the phone. That's probably why I like the solitude."

Van Zee also quickly discovered that two or three hours of cycling weren't enough. He entered road races and then 24-hour events where riders log as many miles as they can on as little sleep as possible. He brought Denise along as his support crew. At first she encouraged him to stop and rest during the rides. "You don't want to do that," he said, smiling. "But after a while she got pretty good."

"The first 24-hour challenge," Denise said, "you think, 'This is insane. This is really dumb.' But pretty soon all of the wives get together, and you start to realize there are a lot of crazy men out here who do this kind of thing."

Denise and Randy have been married for more than 35 years. They have three children, all grown and on their own. Denise works full time as a nursing assistant. She exercises at a wellness center and walks three miles a day. She teaches CPR and is active at church. Many nights, when Van Zee is getting off his bike, she is coming home from a meeting.

"Randy has an inner drive—he's always got to be doing something," she said. "He just plain loves a challenge and I think he finds that in cycling."

Yet she worries about the long-term effects. Some hard-core runners switch to cycling because it is ostensibly easier on the bones. But a 2003 study of masters cyclists at San Diego State University showed that long-distance bicyclists like Van Zee are more susceptible to osteoporosis because the low impact of pedaling does little to toughen up their skeletal system. Sweating also leaches calcium out of their bones.

There have been two cyclists killed in RAAM, in 2003 and 2005. One, Bob Breedlove, was the same age as Van Zee and a fellow Iowan. He was killed in a head-on crash in Colorado. Denise worries about such dangers, but she is more concerned about how beaten her husband gets during the race. "My concern is that he pushes his body so hard," she said. "It takes a terrible toll, and I worry about that."

In the 2004 RAAM, Van Zee's kidneys shut down and he was hospitalized after the race. His hands also paid a terrible price. Nerve damage from constant gripping is a common problem. After he got home, Van Zee couldn't button his shirt and had to use two hands to start the car. Veteran RAAM riders say it could take months before a rider's hands return to normal. It took seven months until his hands no longer felt numb.

Training for RAAM can be all-consuming. Some riders are professional cyclists who are able to devote much of their day to it. Other riders try to keep a semblance of a normal life by logging the necessary bike time but weeding out the extraneous. Former RAAM winner Pete Penseyres, who holds the record for the fastest RAAM crossing, worked full time as a nuclear engineer and still managed to ride 1,000 miles (1,609 km) a week. He believes it is possible to balance work, family, and training—but only if the spouse and children buy into the lifestyle, he says on RAAM's Web site. By his calculations, a rider would have to be on the bike 60 hours a week (riding at an average speed of 16.66 miles per hour) to log 1,000 miles. After working a 45-hour week, getting six hours of sleep a night, and using two hours a day for showering, getting dressed, and eating, Penseyres said he had seven hours of "free" time a week.

Van Zee could not have spent this much time training at his old job. He worked for 27 years at Hope Haven, a religious-based nonprofit organization in northwestern Iowa that provides services for people with disabilities. As Hope Haven grew, so did Van Zee's management responsibilities. He was working 50 to 60 hours a week. "It was constant pressure," he said. "Money was always an issue. My hat goes off to anyone in middle management. They've got the toughest job in the world." In March 2001, he left and went to work for the State of Iowa, although Hope Haven continued to sponsor him. In the 2004 RAAM, he raised more than $13,000, with Hope Haven's help, to refurbish wheelchairs as part of the company's international ministry work.

Van Zee is on the bike even more than Penseyres—closer to 1,150 miles (1,850 km) a week, almost 3,000 hours a year. Cycling has essentially become a second job that constantly demands overtime. "I couldn't do this if my kids were still at home," he said.

Danny Chew, RAAM's winner in 1996 and 1999, believes the ideal age to win RAAM is between 35 and 45. Penseyres was 43 when he recorded the fastest time in the race. "It's really more of a test of will and endurance," said Chew, who analyzes the races online every year. "You have to be in fabulous condition, but you also have to develop good time management in your training," he said. Chew thinks ultramarathon cyclists aren't slowed by age until they reach 45. "In this race, you aren't old until you hit 50," he said.

BIKE, EAT, WORK, EAT, BIKE, AND SLEEP

Van Zee's day begins at 4:00 a.m. when he begins riding on his stationary wind trainer in the basement until an hour or so before daylight. Then he bikes on country roads with the aid of a bike light until 7:30. He showers, eats a quick breakfast, and is at work by 8:00. After work, he takes a short nap and usually has supper with Denise before he is back on the bike at five. He rides until nine o'clock. Iowa winters force him to spend much of his training from November to March indoors. In the basement, he listens to music ("It's got to be uplifting, anything really, from Pink Floyd to Christian rock") and watches old bicycle races. While pedaling, he does isometric exercises for his neck and uses dumbbells for his biceps.

On a weekday, he rides 150 miles (241 km). On Saturdays and Sundays, he rides 200 miles (322 km) a day but makes sure he is home to go out to eat on Saturday night. It's his and Denise's date night.

With all of the riding, Van Zee still thought he wasn't training enough for RAAM 2006. With more than six months to go, he decided to add a third workout every day. By cutting out coffee breaks at work, he left the office at lunch and drove 1.5 miles home and rode the wind trainer for 45 minutes before heading back to work.

After RAAM, Van Zee made a seemingly minor adjustment. In fact, it was a major change for a long-distance cyclist. He began using his large front chain ring, which takes more work to pedal, and his average speed rose 2 miles per hour to a little more than 21 miles per hour (33.7 km per hour) during his training rides. (The average speed of Lance Armstrong's 2005 Tour de France victory was nearly 26 miles per hour, or 41.8 km per hour—and Armstrong often rode in the sanctuary of the peloton; on the other hand, Van Zee doesn't have to contend with mountain stages in Iowa.) Van Zee also increased the amount of weight he was lifting in order to build upper-body strength, and he began visiting a physical therapist to increase his flexibility. The extra work paid off: He was stronger and riding faster than at any other time in his life.

We were having breakfast in Guttenberg when Van Zee's crew members said they noticed that their man had become more buff.

"It was one of the first things I said to Steve when we got in the van," Vaandrager said. "Don't his legs look different? There's more definition this year." Said Moos, "His muscles look longer. He's more solid."

I asked Van Zee if he ever takes a day off.

"I should, but I feel guilty," he said.

"Why?" asks Vaandrager.

She was recruited to join the crew at the urging of Denise, who believed it would help team dynamics if a woman signed on—especially someone like Vaandrager, with her EMT training and a background in physical education. "You need to be obsessed," she told me later. "You need that kind of personality to do RAAM." But she has also been a moderating influence, advocating for Van Zee to dial back, believing it will help in the long run.

Why? The question hangs on him like a hair shirt. It's the question people always ask. Why does he ride so much?

But now it's coming from one of the believers, and the cumulative effects of the long ride and the big breakfast are beginning to take their toll. When he responds to a question, there is a delay, as if he had to think harder about it.

He learned so much the first time around, he told us. The ride was so ugly, so painful. He can do better. The team has learned a lot. The crew will marshal his time better. No more sleeping in hotels. They will have an RV this time. He has a smarter nutrition plan. And even though he's a year older, he is in better condition. He wants to have the fastest time ever for someone over 50—10 days and 6 hours. He tells us that long-distance cycling is deeply woven into his fabric, but he's afraid that if he backs off, everything will start to unravel. "The older you get, the faster your body gets out of shape, and it is harder to get back into shape," he said.

"But don't you think the body needs to rest?" Vaandrager asked.

"Yeah, it does," he said. "I know it does."

"Do you think you are obsessive about it?" she asked.

"Oh, yes, definitely," he said with a sheepish smile. "I have a tendency to overtrain, I know that. But this is more of a positive addiction. I'm pretty organized. I like the routine. It's just become a part of my life."

And to prove his point, he tells us what he describes as his "problem." His in-laws are paying for a Caribbean cruise for the whole family in December to celebrate their 60th wedding anniversary. Van Zee will be on a boat for seven days. There are exercise bikes on board. "But do you think they are going to let me have one for eight hours a day?" he asks. "They'll have to wait in line for me—they'll end up throwing me overboard." (Later, he tells me that he was able to pedal five hours a day in the ship's gym, but he was incredulous that an ocean liner that served food 24 hours a day didn't open their gym until 7:00 a.m.)

At breakfast, our group was fixated on Van Zee. We wanted to know what motivates people who do extraordinary things. But we were surrounded by folks who took their breakfast with smoke and hard liquor, and we ignored an angry man who was blasting billiard balls as if he were shooting grouse.

This is not the kind of crowd who left Oceanside, California, on June 20, 2004, a Sunday morning, for the start of RAAM. There were 19 solo riders, including rookie Randy Van Zee. All of them were men; three were over 50. At the finish in Atlantic City, only eight riders would finish. Even among the riders favored to win, RAAM is as much a personal test as it is a race. The mountains, the heat, the wind, sleep deprivation, calibrating the right mix of food and water, team chemistry, and the riders' health and mental state will conspire against them along the route. Though they start as a group, the race quickly becomes a solitary quest. As cars whizzed by, the contorted faces of passengers scrunched up against the window make the riders' efforts that much more surreal. In the California desert, the temperature hit 113 degrees. By early the second day in the mountain town of Springerville, Arizona, the temperature had fallen to 35. On day 3, the first solo rider dropped out. Three more dropped on day 4 because of problems with knees, strained quads, or saddle sores. By day 5, eight of the riders had quit, but all three of the over-50 riders were still in: Van Zee; Gus Moonen, 52, of the Netherlands; and the oldest soloist, Peter Holy, 57, of Germany.

Van Zee developed stomach problems. His special high-energy liquid diet lasted two days and he began eating cold sandwiches, pasta, pizza, pancakes, and Rice Krispies bars. Saddle sores and Achilles heel problems soon flared up. So did his old hamstring injury. But worse, his neck muscles gave out in New Mexico and he began wearing a bizarre contraption the crew called the "neck wrecker" to give him support to combat the overuse. Van Zee had seen the neck brace in use on a videotape of an old RAAM by former rider and race director Michael Shermer. Just in case he was afflicted by the overuse injury, he showed the tape to two friends who crafted their own neck wrecker. Anchored by a waistband around the torso, the device extended over the top of the helmet like the arm of a crane and pulled his head up high enough so that he could see the road. Without it, with the strength in his neck shot, Van Zee was stooped over like an old man.

The west-to-east orientation takes advantage of the prevailing winds. But Van Zee was battling fierce headwinds on the Great Plains and he was falling behind the pace he set for himself. The finish line was still more than a half a continent away, and he was drowning in a sea of despair. He didn't see how he could make it. In Kansas, in the middle of the night, he got off his bike and threw it into the ditch and buried his head into the hood of his support van. "This is not going to work," he sobbed. The crew gathered around him. His lips were swollen. His faced was sunburned. The race had acted as a virus, probing for weaknesses and then attacking. Everything was in slow motion. His mind was in a fog. He was searching for his glasses and didn't realize they were plastered to his forehead. "Sorry, guys," he mumbled. The crew drove him to a motel and massaged his body while Van Zee slept for three hours.

In Iowa, Denise got a call from Travis Else, the crew chief. She had known something was wrong: RAAM's Web site showed her husband didn't seem to be moving. Friends started a prayer chain. "Northwest Iowa is very churchgoing," she said. "You wouldn't believe the amount of prayer support we got."

The next morning, the team had a meeting. Cheerless gray clouds hung in the air. Else would soon be going back to Michigan to finish his seminary studies. He told Van Zee it was a new day. There would still be plenty of pain ahead, but he asked his rider to rethink the race. The crew would do whatever he wanted, but if Randy decided to keep going, they would get him across. This would be the new starting line. "I said, 'Well, I would really like to finish this thing,'" Van Zee told me. "We weren't going to break any records, but from that point on, there wasn't any question."

Holy, the German, had been trailing Van Zee, but a bad case of saddle sores would force him to drop out in Missouri. Van Zee inherited last place. Danny Chew, the former RAAM winner, determined that Van Zee was slightly ahead of a pace to finish the race within the allotted 12 days and 2 hours. Another racer dropped out ahead of him. Even after his breakdown in Kansas, there were problems. He was still wearing the neck brace. In Ohio, Van Zee fell off his bike, injured his groin, and learned later that he had cracked his pelvis. The crew had to help him get on and off his bike. In West Virginia, he stopped while climbing a mountain, lifted the front wheel, spun the tires, and did the same with the back. "There is something wrong with my bike," he told Else. 'We're going so slow.'"

Else eyed him up and down. "That's because we're going up a very steep hill," he told him. Van Zee looked around.

"Ohhhhhh," he said dreamily and got back on his bike. The crew fell behind with his nutritional supplements, so they doubled the doses. "That's a real no-no," Van Zee told me. He gained 30 pounds of water weight. When he returned to Iowa, he was hospitalized for kidney failure. As Van Zee continued to pedal, the crew grew more worried. Calls were made to doctors back home. They wondered whether they should pull him out of the race. But as he drew closer to the finish, the tide turned. RAAM is a fever chart of emotions, and he began to feel better.

Each morning, the crew laid their hands over him and said a prayer. Vaandrager had nursed his saddle sores, and by the end of the trip they had healed. Others had been stretching his hamstrings and they improved. Cal Helmus, the other crew chief, "was a super motivator for me," Van Zee recalled. "Very positive and encouraging—he kept his head on straight throughout the race."

There was something else that kept him going: For much of RAAM, he was in a race with Moonen, the other 50-something rider. "That helped—a little competition," Van Zee said. "He would pass me, I would pass him, and then at night I would see some flashing lights and that would pick me up and I said, 'I gotta catch that guy.'"

Moonen finished ahead of Van Zee in a time of 11 days, 8 hours, and 9 minutes. He was the seventh rider to complete RAAM.

Van Zee arrived in Atlantic City at 2:40 in the morning to the sound of a few hoots and scattered applause in a time of 11 days, 16 hours, and 26 minutes. He had more than 9 hours to spare before the noon cutoff the next day. The winner, Jure Robic of Slovenia, 39, who became a professional soldier so he could train and race full time, had finished in 8 days, 9 hours, and 51 minutes. Most of the other cyclists, onlookers, and the media had gone home. But Denise and one of their daughters, Rachel, who was living in Germany and whose husband was serving in Iraq, were waiting for him. Van Zee became the 169th solo finisher. More people have climbed to the top of Mount Everest.

Danny Chew, whose life goal is to bicycle 1 million miles, an ambition he won't reach until he is in his mid-70s, believes that Van Zee persevered because he knew his limitations and started out more slowly than others who flamed out along the way. "Nobody looked so bad at the finish line as Randy did," he told me. He awarded Van Zee his unofficial Chew's Most Tired Award for the rider whose body had been beat up the most by RAAM but still managed to finish.

Van Zee could have quit so many times: when his neck gave out in New Mexico, when he fell apart in Kansas, when he crashed in Ohio, or when his kidneys started to fail. Any doctor would have told him that it was only going to get worse. The other riders were all younger. Many were more experienced and better equipped. But Van Zee had reached a stage in his life where he could throw all his energy into a single task. He had

Danny Chew: The Million-Mile Man

Danny Chew's life goal is to ride his bike 1 million miles. By his calculation, he will reach the milestone in 2038, when he turns 75. Until then, his biggest concern isn't whether he will lose his desire. In recent years he has averaged more than 15,000 miles a year. Major injury from riding so much hasn't been a problem, either. What worries him are the cars on the road. Three of his friends have been killed while riding. So far, his closest brush was when he was hit by a deer, knocking him unconscious for 10 hours. Chew was born in 1962. He was the winner of the Race Across America in 1996 and 1999. He has a degree in mathematics from the University of Pittsburgh. He revels in the numbers and statistics of so much riding and has kept detailed accounts since 1978. His first double century—200 miles—was on a Sears Free Spirit when he was 10. He rode his 600,000th mile on September 10, 2006, when he was 44. He rode his millionth kilometer (621,371 miles) on November 24, 2007, at 45. Chew holds no regular job. He lives at home with his mother and supports himself as the statistician and chronicler of Race Across America (RAAM). Chew admits he's addicted to the bike. But it's not like alcohol or cigarettes, because he is exercising as the world around him grows more sedentary. "I like to think of it as a positive addiction," he said.

never done anything harder. He was determined to finish his race across America.

CLOUDS AHEAD

Van Zee told me he never really stopped working out after he got back from Atlantic City in 2004. "I didn't think that I trained hard enough for RAAM the first time," he said. "I think that it was attitude, my mind, that got me through."

So when he came back to Iowa and decided to do RAAM in 2006, he pushed himself harder and got himself into the best shape of his life. It meant rides like the one on the day I met him when he rode nonstop across Iowa. On weekends, he would often leave the house by 4:00 a.m. and ride all day long.

On Saturday, May 20, 2006, a windless day, it took little effort to pedal as he moved across northwestern Iowa at an average speed of 20 miles per hour. By 12:30, he had biked about 160 miles (257 km). Then, extra clothes he had wrapped in a bungee cord on his aerobars unraveled and got caught in the spokes. Van Zee's bike stopped suddenly and flipped over on top of him. He hit the asphalt on the right side of his face. His glasses were smashed. Two of his front teeth were knocked out. He suffered multiple broken bones in his face.

Van Zee never lost consciousness and was able to drag his bicycle off the side of the road. The first motorist didn't have a cell phone. The second did, however, and called 9-1-1. He was taken by ambulance to Orange City three miles away. After X-rays and emergency treatment, Van Zee was transferred 70 miles to Sioux Falls, South Dakota, where he spent the next six days in the hospital.

The broken bones in his face were patched together with titanium plates and screws. His right eye socket had to be reconstructed because doctors thought that his eyeball might fall out. He needed a root canal and bridge work, and some of his teeth had to be ground down to accommodate his newly misaligned jaw. Even over the telephone, months after the accident, he talked as if he had just come back from the dentist. His face was numb from nerve damage, and he has been told it might stay that way the rest of his life.

"The first thing I worried about was RAAM," he said. "I hoped I hadn't blown my chance." RAAM 2006 was out of the question. He was on morphine and his jaw was wired shut. He flirted with the idea anyway, but in the end, he followed the race on the Internet, watching a line on RAAM's Web site move slowly across the country.

I thought the crash would stub out his fire. But the next summer, in August 2007, 55-year-old Van Zee and Bob Thunselle, 49, of Casper, Wyoming, both riding solo and trading leads, shared first place in a 435-mile (700 km) nonstop race across South Dakota called Highway 212 Gut Check. Nineteen solo riders started, but only three finished.

Van Zee started thinking about doing RAAM once more in 2009. He spent the winter of 2007 and early 2008 cycling indoors. On April 4, late on a Friday afternoon, the temperature had climbed into the low 60s and Denise remembered Randy was excited because he had ridden outdoors only twice that spring.

"Have a nice ride," she said before he left.

"Will I ever," he told her.

By 7:15 that night, Van Zee was six miles from Sheldon and heading due west on an isolated stretch of county highway. The east branch of the Floyd River wound through the field on his left, the detritus from last season's grain crop on his right.

The road began to climb. Behind him, a driver in a Pontiac Grand Prix was traveling about 55 miles per hour when she tried passing him. But instead of swinging around, she slammed into him with the right front side of the car. Van Zee struck the bottom of the windshield with the back of his head. He was thrown more than 50 feet, and when he landed on the road, his feet were still clipped into his pedals. Van Zee, who was wearing a helmet, suffered head and leg injuries and was pronounced dead at the scene. He was 56.

"I am sure that he was having his thoughts for the day and didn't even know it when he was struck," Sergeant Brad Krei of the Iowa State Patrol told me.

It had been a bright, glorious day and the sun at the time of the accident had been low in the sky. But Trooper John Skaar, an accident investigator with the state patrol, didn't think the conditions would have blinded the driver. He went back to the scene a couple of days later, at the same time, when the sun was again shining, and concluded that the sun played no role in the accident. The motorist, a 21-year-old woman, was ticketed for not having car insurance and failing to stop at a safe distance, according to the accident report. Skaar checked Van Zee's bike computer and found that he had ridden 30 miles.

Three weeks later, I called Denise. I had written her after the accident and told her that I thought that Randy was someone who would ride forever.

"I do miss him terribly," she said. Even though cycling blogs and a blog from a local newspaper resurrected in the public eye the uneasy relationship between bicycle riders and motorists, Denise told me she called the young driver and told her she knew it was an accident and was praying for her. She also didn't blame Randy for upping the odds by riding so much. That spring, the couple's youngest daughter, Rachel Carlson, a young mother and wife of an army officer who was bound for his second tour of Iraq, was training for a triathlon. She and Randy were a lot alike. When she was still home, they were the ones who took care of the family's dogs, wolf hybrids, and took them on long walks. Training for races stoked their competitive nature and provided periods of solitude—Randy liked to call it reflection—that they craved so much. When Rachel came home from Colorado for the funeral, she told Denise she was thinking about not entering the race. Maybe it would be best to lay off for a while.

"You know what your dad would want," Denise told her. "Get back on the bike."

12

Marathon Man

A sea of hands shot into the air when the runners were asked how many of them had ever finished 10 marathons.

Twenty? A hundred?

The crowd at the spaghetti dinner the night before the 2005 Quad Cities Marathon started looking around to see who among them had run so far, so many times. Two hundred? Finally, the hands of only two men remained raised.

One was Ray Scharenbrock (born in 1933), a retired teacher from South Milwaukee, Wisconsin. He was 72 years old and had run 506 marathons.

At the same table was Don McNelly (born in 1920) of Rochester, New York. McNelly was 84. With his white beard and protruding belly, he bore more of a passing resemblance to Santa Claus than a dyed-in-the-wool runner. He had run or walked 679 marathons.

The Quad Cities crowd applauded. They understood the pain and the pleasure of running so many marathons over so many years. There are many motivations for running a marathon. It can simply be a life goal. It can serve as a benchmark for personal fitness. It can be an inward journey in a frenetic world. Some enter a marathon to raise money for a good cause. Others take a lighter view of it all and see the 26.2 miles as a rolling, undulating party where the drinking and eating start at the end. Whatever a runner's motivation, it remains the most famous benchmark of endurance in the world.

Earlier in the day I had scanned the Quad Cities entrant list and found that baby boomers made up the lion's share of the runners. But when I tried to find contemporaries of McNelly, there weren't any. I found no runners in their 80s. I found only one runner in his 70s. (Scharenbrock had entered the half marathon.) When I got to people in their 60s, I counted 19.

McNelly was entering two marathons a month, often flying great distances to do it. The next week, he ran a marathon in Japan where he was a member of local running society. He was the oldest and slowest member and the only one with a size 15 shoe. From there, he stopped in Portland, Oregon, for another marathon and to indulge in another pastime. McNelly is an elephant buff, and he attended a national meeting of elephant handlers.

The rigor of so many marathons and so much travel is at times tiring for McNelly. But each completed race is also an affirmation of good health and a good life. A retired business executive, he has the financial wherewithal to continue, and it keeps him connected to a vast social network. At each event he not only chalks up another marathon; he is also recognized, even lionized, for his accomplishments.

By 4:30 the next morning I was in my car following McNelly and a running acquaintance, Jill Vorwald, as they were driven across the Mississippi River from Moline, Illinois, to Bettendorf, Iowa, for the start of the marathon.

The rest of the runners would leave the starting line in Moline at 7:30. The marathon starts in Illinois, crosses the river into Iowa, and returns to Illinois. The final blocks in Moline would be lined with cheering spectators. But because he was walking the course, McNelly needed an early start so he could finish before the six-hour time limit elapsed. At this time of the morning, the bridge over the Mississippi on Interstate 74 was closed to pedestrians, so McNelly and Vorwald started out ahead and made up the two miles by retracing their steps later in the race. His mind, he told me, "goes into a neutral, kind of a funk. It's a free flow of thoughts that I really enjoy."

With flashlight in hand and a handkerchief tucked into his cap for sun protection, they began walking down one dark and cheerless street after another. I stayed with them for a few miles. When I left, they were chatting amiably until they faded from sight.

This was not a run in the fast lane. They would finish in 8:46:12—about twice as slow as the median time for a male marathon runner. There are certainly faster aging marathoners. Ed Whitlock, a whippet-thin Canadian, ran an astounding world-record 3:04:54 at the age of 76 in Rotterdam in 2007. Fauja Singh was 92 when he set an equally impressive world record for nonagenarians in a Toronto marathon in a time of 5:40:01.

MARATHON RANKS SWELL

The number of marathon finishers has risen from 143,000 in 1980 to 412,000 in 2007, according to Running USA's Road Running Information Center. The growth has been fueled, in part, by promoters who are marketing their marathons as vehicles for charitable causes and for their entertainment value as much as for tests of endurance.

The increase in numbers has slowed the average marathon time. Runners who were content to stick with a shorter distance are more quickly graduating to the marathon. The median finishing time of men has slowed from 3:32:17 in 1980 to 4:15:34 in 2006. Women's times have slowed from 4:03:39 to 4:46:40, according to Running USA, a nonprofit organization dedicated to promoting running.

McNelly is a member of a pair of running clubs where time is incidental. Members of the 50 States Marathon Club try to knock off a marathon in every state. The 50 States & D.C. Marathon Group USA adds a marathon in the District of Columbia. The 50-staters are a culture within a subculture. They seek each other out, trade stories, and critique the layout of a marathon course much as itinerant golfers do.

Sometimes they knock off states with their own peculiar twist. Scharenbrock had run marathons or ultramarathons in all of the states and D.C. *eight* times when we met in the Quad Cities. When I caught up with him in late 2008, he had finished his 9th circuit and was nearly done with his 10th. No one has done more marathon circuits than Scharenbrock. The Quad Cities Half Marathon in 2005 had counted toward a new goal: being the first person to run half marathons in every state and D.C. He knocked that off a year later. Scharenbrock, 75, fully expects the younger generation to surpass him. He seemed resigned to it. "The great men say that records are made to be broken," he said.

One of McNelly's closest friends, Wally Herman of Ottawa, Canada, was the first runner to complete a marathon in all 50 states, plus D.C. He reached that goal in 1983, but it took him until 1985 to run marathons in all the Canadian provinces because his wedding anniversary coincided with a must-do marathon in the Yukon. "It took me a few years to extract myself from my wife to do that one," he told me in a conspiratorial voice. Herman holds the record for the most marathons in foreign countries. He's run marathons in 99 countries, according to 50 States & D.C. Marathon Group USA.

McNelly has also run marathons in all states plus D.C. He is ranked third in America in total marathons. His stop in the 2005 Quad Cities Marathon brought his total to 680. The top megamarathoner in North America is his friend, Norm Frank, a fellow resident of Rochester. He is 10 years younger than McNelly and at the time was closing in on 900 marathons.

McNelly has no aspirations of moving up. His specialty is that he's finished more marathons after the age of 70 than anyone else in the world. Quad Cities would be his 409th marathon after turning 70.

"I claim it as a world record," he said. "And I've yet to hear from anyone to dispute it."

A POSITIVE ADDICTION

Thom Gilligan, the operator of Marathon Tours & Travel in Boston, said that McNelly is the prototype of a generation of men who were successful in their careers and needed goals to feed their fire. He thinks that McNelly is addicted to the challenge of piling up an ever-growing mountain of marathon finishes.

Gilligan stages a marathon in Antarctica, which McNelly ran. Two kinds of people are attracted to such trips: boomers who need something outside of their work to feed their ego and retired men and women looking for another novel piece of real estate on which to run a marathon. "At some point when you get older, you hate to give up, because otherwise you are giving up on yourself," Gilligan said. "I think they love it and it keeps their adrenaline going."

Phyllis McNelly, Don's wife of 66 years, has lived with it since her husband began running in his 50s. "I think that it's a little excessive," she told me in the fall of 2007. The couple has two sons, a statistician and a designer of computer chips. Their daughter, a medical researcher, died in 2004 at 55 of a mysterious heart ailment. "I think that Dr. Cooper once told Don that if you run for more than 30 minutes at a time, you are running for something more than your health," Phyllis said.

Dr. Cooper is Kenneth H. Cooper, the Dallas physician who helped fuel the running boom with his best-selling book *Aerobics*. Like Clarence Bass and thousands of other men and women, McNelly has made periodic visits to the Cooper Clinic for an assessment of his physical condition and vindication that all of the sweating is paying off.

"I *am* addicted to it," he told me. "But I hasten to add that it's a positive addiction."

McNelly has not been immune to the effects of aging. In 1989, he had his prostate removed after cancer was found. He broke three ribs falling off a ladder in 1996. In 2000, he had surgery to remove a benign growth near his spine. He has had plantar fasciitis, a common overuse injury that causes pain on the heel and the sole of the foot. He also has suffered from inflamed metatarsals on both feet. After he turned 80, his cardiologist found some blockage in the arteries around his heart. He takes medication for elevated blood pressure and cholesterol levels. He has also undergone surgery on his upper lip for skin cancer.

But at our first meeting in 2005, he looked much younger than 84. When he got up from a chair in his hotel room to pour us a cup of coffee, he moved lightly across the room. There was no unsteady movement, no big production getting out of the chair. His resting heart rate was 48 beats a minute.

The Cooper Clinic

Dr. Kenneth H. Cooper began assessing patients in 1970 after the popular success of his 1968 book *Aerobics*. The clinic has examined nearly 100,000 people since then.

Cooper believes people should exercise 30 minutes a day on most days. His philosophy is that as you age, the proportion of aerobic exercise should fall and the amount of weight training should increase to ameliorate the weakening of bone and muscle over time. In your 30s, he recommends 80 percent aerobics and 20 percent weight training; in your 40s, it's 70 and 30 percent; in your 50s, it's 60 and 40 percent; at 60 and older, it's 55 percent aerobics and 45 percent weight training.

The core service at the clinic is a comprehensive medical examination and preventive medicine counseling, which includes an electrocardiogram and stress tests on a treadmill or stationary bicycle. Services can range from $2,800 to $5,000.

Had McNelly, who is 6-foot-1 and weighs 210 pounds (185 cm, 95 kg), been a speed demon in his younger days, or even in middle age, he thinks he would have gotten sick of running or worn his body down. In his 50s, he joined a running group in Rochester, but all of the others have dropped out. Physically, they couldn't run any longer or couldn't cope with going slower.

"The people who destroyed themselves were the really thin people—they bust their asses every time they go out," he said. "They pull muscles and knees go bad. Then they quit running. They let their egos get in the way. They're like football players. Twenty years after their prime, they are hobbling around. They are beat up. They paid for it later."

"I feel blessed. I am very fortunate to be able to do this. I was never fast, so I never got caught up in that supercompetitiveness. I never killed myself to set a new PR. And I never got caught in the age-group thing because I am so old."

He smiled. "I nearly always win an age group," he said. "I don't even have to try."

FIRST MARATHON AT 48

McNelly, a retired vice president of St. Joe Co., a paper, timber, and real estate company headquartered in Jacksonville, Florida, started running after a friend dropped dead of a heart attack. "Those were the days when guys were eating steaks and drinking martinis, and I was one of them," he said. His doctor told him to lose weight and get some exercise. The doctor was running three miles a day, "so he had credibility," McNelly said. The doctor also recommended that he read Cooper's best-seller.

"I got the book and read it, and he said in there that if you get yourself in shape, with proper conditioning, your average (resting) heart rate will drop 10 beats a minute," McNelly recalled. "That's 14,400 beats a day. I still remember those numbers. You figure, if God gave you so many heartbeats, you can extend your life. That did it. It sold me."

At the age of 48 he ran his first race, the 1969 Boston Marathon, nine months after he started running. He made a beginner's mistake and went out too fast and was forced to start walking after four miles. He finished in 5:01. Boston had 1,342 entrants that year, and when he went back to work, the concept of distance running was so novel, "I was a hero in the company," he said.

Although McNelly has a wide array of interests, long-distance running became his chief hobby. In 1975, at the age of 54, McNelly and four brothers (two of them smokers) set a world record for a family in a relay by running 133 miles, 1,320 yards (215.2 km) in 24 hours. McNelly ran 27 miles; his brothers ran about the same. A few weeks later, he took part in another 24-hour relay with nine other men. That time they set a record for runners 50 and over.

In 1982, at the age of 61, he and 15 other men between the ages of 50 and 61 took part in a relay run across the United States to raise $35,000 for a children's hospital in Rochester, where McNelly still serves on the board. Living out of a pair of motor homes, the runners took only two showers over the 17-day crossing. McNelly remembered the brilliant skies at night and the depression he felt on the third night when the immensity of what lay ahead seemed overwhelming. He battled pneumonia all the way. The hardest section was going up the Rockies near Steamboat Springs, Colorado; the most rewarding was passing through his hometown of Clayton, Ohio, where family and old friends, 53 in all, met them at midnight for coffee and doughnuts "to watch the idiots run by," he said.

In 1983, to promote the Empire State Games, he and a group of runners from Rochester zigzagged 1,000 miles (1,609 km) from Shea Stadium to Syracuse. McNelly got to light the flame at the opening of the Games. "The number-one thrill of my life," he said.

McNelly is an engineer by training. But he has a salesman's heart. "He's an upbeat guy," said Wally Herman. "He doesn't have a negative bone in his body."

For someone drawn to such an individual sport, McNelly revels in the company of others. "You have to be comfortable with yourself when you run," he said. "You have to be willing to be a loner—or at least, in my case, a gregarious loner."

He also has a knack for telling a tale. One of his hardest marathons was Thom Gilligan's tour to Antarctica. He had to traverse glaciers and cross icy streams. What the route lacked in cheering throngs it made up for in waddling penguins. "Penguins are not an endangered species—and you can quote me on that," he said.

Once, he led a blind runner, a college professor from North Carolina, over a gravel road that served as the course of a marathon on Baffin Island, almost 500 miles (804 km) north of the Arctic Circle. When they finished, the man's wife turned him around and the couple ran another marathon back to the start.

He has run the marathon in Nanisivik, Nunavut, formerly a part of the Northwest Territories, 13 times. "It's so far up north that if you can get away from other people—from other runners—it is the quietest place I have ever been in my life," he said. "There is no noise. No color, except blue sky."

He's done a marathon even farther to the north, a desolate expanse ringed by mountains, in Spitzbergen, Norway, which is billed as the northernmost marathon in the world. He's run marathons in Greenland twice and Iceland once. He has run the Boston Marathon 30 times (28 times as a bandit because he wasn't fast enough to make the qualifying time) and finished all of the other majors in the United States. He's run up the Empire State Building. He brought along Phyllis when he ran marathons in Paris, London, and Rotterdam on three successive weekends—much of the trip paid by a friend, a fellow runner, as a gift for the couple's 50th wedding anniversary.

In Panama, he's run 50-mile races on two occasions. Both of them took place at night when it was cooler. Each runner was followed by a driver who used his headlights to light the course. The heat and humidity made him woozier than a typical marathon would. "The hardest thing I ever did in my life," he said.

For nearly all of these runs he has given me copies of newspaper clippings and other records. McNelly is keenly aware that he participates in a form of running that requires honor among its practitioners. At each event, he tries to make sure that he sees someone who can affirm that he was there. The universe of megamarathoners is relatively small, and McNelly invariably runs into someone he knows.

We got together for a second time in Moline for the Quad Cities Marathon in September 2007. In November he would turn 87. Though McNelly started running marathons nearly as soon as he took up the sport, his most impressive statistic is the number he has run late in life.

"Don didn't start running until our family was pretty well raised, and I think that should sort of be a warning for young runners with small children," Phyllis told me. "They shouldn't get too hooked on running until their children don't need as much help on the weekends. When Don retired, he had been so busy that the family wondered how he was going to keep active. He was doing volunteer work. But he had discovered running and he starting spending more time on that. We never worried about what he was going to do ever since."

In the fall of 2007, he had run or walked 455 marathons after the age of 70. He had finished 159 marathons after turning 80. He was coming up to 59,000 miles (94,951 km) of marathons and ultramarathons since he took up the sport. We leafed through spreadsheets he updates on his computer to show me what he thinks is his best stat: Since he turned 85 he had finished 42 marathons.

"This is the one that amazes me," he said, smiling and clearly pleased. "How in the hell can anyone do that? You've got to be *alive*. You've got to make it to 85. How many people do you know who are even alive at 85? I am proud of that one."

McNelly also keeps track of his expenses for entering and traveling to races. Since 1990, his figures show that he had spent $149,648 after counting Quad Cities. The figure is conservative, he said, because if he mixes the trip with a vacation, or if Phyllis comes along, he subtracts that part of the expense.

In addition to serving on the board of the children's hospital, which is part of the University of Rochester Medical Center, McNelly is a board member at the Seneca Park Zoo Society in Rochester. His affiliation with the zoo got McNelly interested in elephants. He's attended an elephant-handling school and once, on behalf of the zoo, carried a vial of elephant semen on a plane back home. He also makes wine, and he is an amateur historian. He's sent me articles he has written, such as "One Thousand Years of Military Elephants" and "A Short History of the Second Most Famous Elephant in North America." When we met in 2007, he was working on a piece about typhoons that destroyed U.S. naval ships in World War II in the South Pacific, where he served.

Before arriving in Illinois, McNelly had left Rochester and driven in his Toyota Corolla to Austin, Texas, to visit one of his sons. Then he traveled to Fredericksburg, Texas, to the National Museum of the Pacific War to attend a symposium on Guadalcanal and the Battle of Midway. From there he drove to Kansas City to visit an old friend before arriving in the Quad Cities.

McNelly's sheer doggedness is a celebration of his longevity. But the data contained in his spreadsheets are a grim reminder that he is slowing down. Each year, he takes his 10 best times and averages them. In 1990, at age 70, his times averaged 4:35:00, or about a 10:30-per-mile pace. By 2006, the times had increased to 8:30:00, or nearly a 20-minute pace.

He started walking marathons at about age 80. At first he was embarrassed by it. But he wasn't surprised because his decline became apparent at 74. That year, his average best times fell by nearly a half hour. "You get older and things begin to fall apart," he said.

McNelly was the subject of a longitudinal study by gerontologists at the University of Maryland's School of Medicine and the Baltimore Veteran Medical Affairs Medical Center. In the study (published in 2003 in the *American Journal of Cardiology*), researchers examined his aerobic capacity over 12 years and found that his maximum rate of oxygen consumption fell 44 percent between the ages of 68 and 80. But his weekly mileage had fallen off only 10 percent during the period. He was walking slower, but he kept piling on the miles.

McNelly thinks that he could push his times down for a year or two, "but then it would slip right back," he told me as we sitting in his hotel room.

There was a knock on the door, and in walked Jim Reeve. He is another megamarathoner. He and McNelly were sharing a room the night before the 2007 Quad Cities Marathon. Reeve was 65 at the time and retired and living in South Padre Island, Texas. He had completed 567 marathons. In 1980, when he was 48, he ran 63 marathons in 12 months.

The two of them traded stories about their brethren, including running legend Ed Barreto, a Floridian who ran 84 marathons in 52 weeks and played a single down for the Ashland (Ohio) University football team when he was 60. "He's even crazier than us," Reeve said.

McNelly said runners are already drawing a bead on his marathon tally, and he thinks a baby boomer will break his totals for marathons after 70 and 80. "Oh, they're going to do it," he said. "I know because people are already calling me. They're already trying. It's easier to break a goal than to set a goal because it's out there."

McNelly looked over at Reeve, 20 years younger. "In his heart of hearts, he thinks he is going to catch me," McNelly said.

"Don has an ego that pushes him along," observed his friend Wally Herman. "He is interested in having that big marathon number."

McNelly won't dispute it. "I get an awful lot of satisfaction about being the oldest finisher," he said. Runners wait around for McNelly to finish to tell him they hope to be doing same thing. "That means an awful lot to me," he said.

A SETBACK

In the morning, McNelly and Jill Vorwald were once again getting a ride across the Mississippi from Vorwald's sister, Judy. This year, the entourage included Reeve and me. By 5:00, we started to walk. McNelly had driven 3,000 miles (4,830 km) on this trip, and his left knee was hurting. He wasn't sure it would hold up. The night before at dinner, I noticed he had trouble getting out of the booth.

But there were bigger problems. Earlier in the summer, McNelly had finished two months of radiation—38 treatments in all—to kill cancer cells that had returned to where his prostate had been removed. He had finished nine marathons in 2007, but he had completed only two since the last of his radiation treatments. Two weeks earlier in Pennsylvania at the windy and rain-soaked Erie Marathon at Presque Isle, he quit after six miles.

As we started from Bettendorf, the temperature was in the mid-50s. The stars glistened in the night sky. Our pace was slow. McNelly was clearly not the man I met two years earlier—a fact corroborated by Vorwald. The two of them met at the marathon in 1999, and it wasn't until the final miles on the course that he told her about the hundreds of marathons that he had completed. They've done Quad Cities together most years since then.

"We never walked at this pace," she said.

We moved on, and when the sun rose, it lifted everybody's spirits. McNelly told me that his last stop on the way home would be Chicago,

An Octogenarian's Perspective

Marathons are much better organized than when Don McNelly started running them in 1969. Courses then weren't as well marked. Marathons had only minimal supervision, so runners had to keep their eyes peeled for stoplights and railroad crossings. "You were kind of on your own out there," McNelly said. The sport changed in 1972 after Frank Shorter won the gold medal in the Olympics. It gave marathons a big boost. But as their popularity has grown, their exalted status has diminished a bit—and McNelly misses that. When he started, the oldest age-group classification was 40—he was 48 at the time. Age groups kept rising, but he always found himself at the old end of new brackets. Now age divisions rarely go higher than 70. He'd like to see race directors add 5-year increments after 70. McNelly, who walks marathons now, thinks some of his contemporaries grew frustrated when their times slowed, so they dropped out. He believes it's more important to keep going.

where he would visit the Lincoln Park Zoo and have dinner with the urologist who had operated on him 18 years ago.

At the 12-mile mark, McNelly said he was getting tired. I wasn't quite sure what to make of it because I had never done a marathon before. My hamstrings and lower back were beginning to get sore, and I had to stop and stretch. So far, the marathon hadn't seemed anything like a race. It was a leisurely, albeit long, walk. We strolled through a historic section of Rock Island, drifting from one conversation to the next. McNelly, though laboring at times, seemed to be having a good time. Relay teams that would run sections of the course were beginning to assemble, and several bands were starting to tune up for the runners who were closing in on us.

We crossed another bridge to Arsenal Island, home of a sprawling government-owned weapons manufacturing facility. Our route wound mostly through a golf course and passed a warren of 19th- and early-20th-century homes that had been built for officers. The leaders of the half marathon began passing us, and shortly afterward, the lead marathoner, a Kenyan, flew by. The speed of the runners and the constant pitter-pat of footsteps seemed jarring after having the course to ourselves for so many hours.

We were now in the middle of it all; runners of all sizes and running styles were passing us. Reeve left us and started walking with a fellow Texan. McNelly spit a lot. Vorwald, who was 48, married, and the mother of two teenage boys, talked almost nonstop. Her family lives in the country near Dubuque, Iowa. Her monologue on local happenings, the lives of her sons, and her wandering, sexually active Labradors kept our minds off the long grind.

"McNelly!" yelled Lois Berkowitz, a founder of the 50 States Marathon Club, who walked by us. "Good job!"

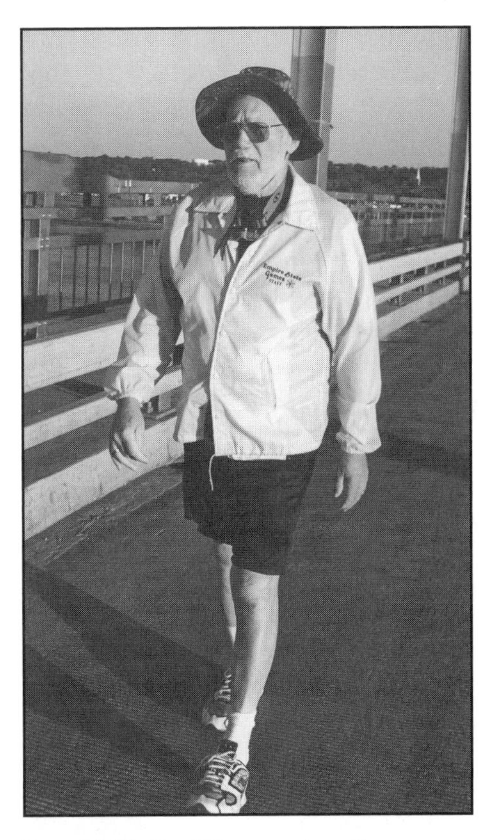

Don McNelly, 86, crossing the Mississippi River at the 2007 Quad Cities Marathon.

Another runner called out and told McNelly he was a legend. He waves back. "I love it!" he said. "I love it!"

At the 18th mile, he took a couple of Tylenol capsules. His knee, which he feared would be his downfall, seemed to be fine. But the rest of his body was hurting, and he told me now that he thought the general effects of age and the radiation treatments were taking their toll. We were coming up on the 20th mile—for us, it was really the 17th because of our early start across the bridge. It was there that the course swung by McNelly's hotel. He would stop there.

I really wanted him to finish. But as Vorwald and I continued on, and the hours of walking began to take its toll on us, I started coming to my senses. McNelly was nearing his 87th birthday. He was fighting cancer for a second time. He had just driven 3,000 miles and then walked 17 miles. The temperature was 90 degrees. A lot of people were walking. Most were 30 or 40 years younger. A few weeks later, under only slightly warmer conditions, a runner would die at the Chicago Marathon.

I had asked McNelly earlier if he ever thought about stopping, especially in light of the cancer. "I think I am coming back," he said. "I think some of it is mental. You lose a little confidence in yourself."

A year later he told me he was running fewer marathons. Flying was becoming more of a hassle, and he was driving more—and farther—to make races. As of January 1, 2009, he had finished 741 marathons.

"Someday, I know that I am going to have to stop," he told me after Quad Cities. "I understand that. I'm not going to go forever. But I am going to keep at it as long as I can."

Epilogue

Ageless Role Models

Let me introduce one final athlete. Payton Jordan is a former track coach at Stanford University who coached the Olympic team in Mexico City in 1968. He was a sprint star in college and was featured on the cover of *Life* magazine in 1939. Then came World War II, and afterward, he turned his attention to teaching and coaching. He didn't compete again until he was 55. When he came back, he remained a champion into his 80s.

We'd talk on the phone occasionally. But more often, I would receive wonderfully upbeat letters with neatly folded news clippings about his career. In one letter, he enclosed a copy of a speech he gave in Los Angeles where he told the audience, "We don't get old. We grow old. If we think of aging as a disease, life will be tough because we cannot cure aging. But we can hold it back."

At 84, he retired from competitive track. His wife needed him more and Jordan's health was deteriorating. Over the next few years he would suffer through two bouts of cancer.

We finally met in 2006 at his apartment in a Santa Barbara, California, retirement center. He was 89. By then, Marge was very sick and would not live much longer. As we talked, he was clearly preoccupied with her care.

Still, Jordan was staying active. As he was giving me a tour, he moved so quickly I nearly had to jog to keep up. He no longer sprinted but preferred walking and lifting weights. In the gym, he plopped down on the leg-press machine, set it at 400 pounds, and began pumping his legs. "I like to explode," he said after getting up. "I want to activate those fast-nerve impulses. I want to be quick and fast."

It wasn't Jordan's preponderance of fast-twitch muscles that kept him in such remarkable condition. He simply loved pushing himself. His joy transcended the mechanical aspects of exercise. He explained this to me in one of our early conversations, just as he was realizing he would probably never race again.

"You run almost ethereally when you run well," he said. "It's almost like a beautiful piece of music. You can't explain why it sounds so good, but it does. You can't say why this piece of literature reads so well, but it does. I wanted running to be a piece of art. You look at a painting and it hits you right between the eyes. When I am running well, when I see someone running well, that's what happens to me I see that. I feel that. I sense it. I live it. That's what it's all about."

Few older athletes can match Jordan's eloquence, but many fully understand the deeper meaning of human movement and are driven by it. Obviously, it makes them feel better. But they've also found an intrinsic good in sweat. Philippa Raschker's ambition helped her find new ways to train when her body began to wear out. Randy Van Zee's obsessive streak caused him untold pain, but it also drove him to quit smoking and switch to a sport that ostensibly would cause fewer injuries. Greg Osterman's heart transplant was an epiphany that opened the door to a healthy lifestyle. Had his heart not failed, he would have remained a hard-drinking plumber. Barb Klippel used old-fashioned goal setting to overcome cancer and a broken skull to become the oldest woman to ski the American Birkebeiner. Octogenarian Don McNelly keeps knocking off marathons to rub shoulders with old friends and accept the inevitable praise for his astounding longevity.

All of this may seem too much to some—especially since health experts tell us that 30 minutes of exercise five days a week is enough. So I found it ironic that Clarence Bass' quest for physical perfection revolved around a commonsense regimen of weight training twice a week, aerobic exercise twice a week, and lots of walks. I think Trip Hedrick became a faster swimmer in middle age because he started late and feels he has to catch up. Did you once dream of greatness beneath a street light in a summer game of tag? I think it's why we can identify with Thom Weisel's ambition to become a champion age-group cyclist and Gail Roper's drive to keep breaking new records in the pool.

The experiences of these men and women aren't so different from our own. The human body is a wonderful engine. And it wants to be pushed.

Appendix

Official USRSA Streak Registries

Official List of Active U.S. Running Streaks (as certified by the United States Running Streak Association, December 1, 2008)

		Start date	Hometown, occupation, age
The Legend (40+ years)			
1.	Mark Covert	07/23/68	Lancaster, CA, teacher and coach, 58
The Grand Masters (35+ years)			
2.	Jon Sutherland	05/26/69	West Hills, CA, writer, 58
3.	Jim Pearson	02/16/70	Ferndale, WA, retiree, 64
4.	Kenneth C. Young	07/06/70	Petrolia, CA, software developer, 67
5.	Stephen W. DeBoer	06/07/71	Rochester, MN, dietitian, 54
6.	Jon A. Simpson	08/30/71	Memphis, TN, dentist, 70
7.	Alex T. Galbraith	12/22/71	Houston, TX, attorney, 58
8.	David L. Hamilton	08/14/72	Portland, OR, sales, 54
9.	Steven Gathje	09/25/72	Overland Park, KS, actuary, 53
The Masters (30+ years)			
10.	Walter O. Byerly	11/05/74	Dallas, TX, real estate agent, 78
11.	Robert R. Kraft	01/01/75	Miami Beach, FL, songwriter, 58
12.	Dick Vincent	03/19/75	Palenville, NY, sales representative, 56

(continued)

The Masters (30+ years) *(continued)*			
13T.	Stephen D. Reed	06/16/76	Wiscasset, ME, doctor, 60
13T.	Robert J. Zarambo	06/16/76	Whitehall, PA, retiree, 61
15.	William S. Stark	09/10/76	St. Louis, MO, professor, 61
16.	Bill Anderson	09/27/76	Fort Worth, TX, retiree, 63
17.	John Liepa	01/02/77	Indianola, IA, professor, 63
18.	Bill Robertson	02/08/77	Ashland, MA, systems analyst, 56
19.	William J. Benton	04/23/77	Farmington Hills, MI, accountant, 58 *
20.	Brian Casey	05/09/77	Paramus, NJ, finance manager, 50
21.	Joseph J. Wojcik	06/13/77	Claremont, CA, retiree, 67
22.	Samuel F. Johnston	08/26/77	Naples, FL, retiree, 66
23.	John T. Carlson	12/26/77	Indianapolis, IN, athletic director, 54
24.	Timothy C. Masters	12/28/77	Dearborn, MI, sales, 58
25T.	Charles Brumley	01/01/78	Saranac Lake, NY, retiree, 69
25T.	Barry Abrahams	01/01/78	Lincoln, NE, teacher, 57 *
27.	Timothy Woodbridge	03/05/78	Allentown, PA, banker, 51
28.	Bruce A. Sherman	05/16/78	Shaker Heights, OH, exercise physiologist, 53
29.	Julie A. Maxwell	07/05/78	Kasson, MN, attorney, 57
30.	C. David Todd	10/14/78	Matthews, NC, home builder, 56
31.	Charles Lindsey	10/16/78	Canyon Country, CA, educator, 57
32.	Harvey B. Simon	10/31/78	Newton, MA, physician, 66
33.	John C. Roemer, IV	11/01/78	Parkton, MD, consultant, 48
34.	Craig A. Davidson	11/05/78	Phoenix, AZ, retail/educator, 54
35.	Scott Ludwig	11/30/78	Peachtree City, GA, operations manager, 53
The Dominators (25+ years)			
36.	Chester A. Tumidajewicz	12/25/78	Amsterdam, NY, security supervisor, 54
37.	Jon Kralovic	01/01/79	Delanson, NY, college football coach, 62
38.	Charles Holmberg	03/20/79	Modesto, CA, CEO, 60
39.	John W. Morgan	04/29/79	Emmett, ID, business owner, 67
40.	Margaret O. Blackstock	09/09/79	Atlanta, GA, homemaker, 64
41.	Dwight A. Moberg	10/06/79	Manhattan Beach, CA, retiree, 76
42.	Bill Beach	10/28/79	Macomb, MI, teacher, 60
43.	Benjamin M. Freed	12/12/79	Clarion, PA, college teacher, 61
44.	S. Mark Courtney	12/20/79	Grove City, PA, physician's assistant, 52
45T.	Layne C. Party	01/01/80	Towson, MD, manager, 49
45T.	William G. Finkbeiner	01/01/80	Auburn, CA, landscaper, 52
47.	William A. Etter	04/08/80	Ferndale, CA, woodworker, 66

48.	Leslie J. Shoop	04/28/80	Saxonburg, PA, retiree, 60
49.	Ed Goff	08/13/80	Bradenton, FL, teacher, 65
50.	John I. Watts	10/04/80	Bend, OR, church superintendent, 53
51.	Ward D. Crutcher	12/26/80	Muncie, IN, retiree, 69
52.	Brian P. Short	12/27/80	Minneapolis, MN, CEO, 58
53.	George G. Brown	01/06/81	Richlands, VA, school principal, 56
54.	Joseph J. Sinicrope	04/22/81	East Granby, CT, retiree, 66
55.	John R. Chandler	08/09/81	Whitefish Bay, WI, financial planner, 53
56.	Steven R. Morrow	08/10/81	Eagle Lake, MN, software engineer, 45
57.	Ben Dillow	08/20/81	Redlands, CA, retiree, 68
58.	Bill Leibfritz	12/03/81	Midland, MI, professor, 52
59.	Frederick L. Murolo	12/30/81	Cheshire, CT, attorney, 51
60.	Scott D. Snyder	12/31/81	Littleton, CO, emergency physician, 53
61.	William Moreland, Jr.	01/15/82	Ocean City, NJ, educator, 62
62.	Michael G. Sklar	01/20/82	Dunwoody, GA, professor, 65
63.	Bob Kimball	02/03/82	Pensacola, FL, professor, 65
64.	Ken Birse	04/22/82	Amherst, NH, data sales manager, 48
65.	Grant McAllister	08/28/82	Atlanta, GA, sales manager, 45
66.	Kenneth D. Korosec	10/16/82	Chesterland, OH, attorney, 64
67.	John J. Strumsky, Jr.	05/23/83	Millersville, MD, writer, 68
68.	Gary Rust	07/03/83	Palm Springs, CA, executive director, 62
69.	Doug Holland	08/01/83	Tucson, AZ, college athletic director, 47
The Highly Skilled (20+ years)			
70.	Paul N. Christian	09/21/84	Rochester, MN, news reporter, 58
71.	Lou Galipeau	01/01/85	Huntsville, AL, sales manager, 63
72.	Leonard Bruckman	02/10/85	Granite Bay, CA, business owner, 61
73.	Bill Bonarrigo	02/20/85	Parkville, MD, manager, 68
74.	Timothy M. Osberg	06/04/85	Grand Island, NY, professor, 53
75.	Matthew A. Mace	09/29/85	Arnold, MD, attorney, 48
76.	Kenneth D. Brown	11/10/85	Huntington, WV, farmer, 59
77.	Ralph McKinney	01/01/86	Wilmington, DE, consultant, 63
78.	William C. Terrell	09/14/86	LaGrange, GA, senior director, 59
79.	John Metevia	10/19/86	Midland, MI, small business owner, 51
80.	Stuart X. Calderwood	01/21/87	New York, NY, writer, 50
81.	Robert E. Nash	06/18/87	Olney, IL, physician, 61
82.	Roger B. Carlson	01/01/88	Stillwater, MN, retiree, 65
83.	Tom Allen	05/21/88	Upper Montclair, NJ, consultant, 56
84.	George M. Church	07/30/88	Cockeysville, MD, attorney, 61

(continued)

Official List of Active U.S. Running Streaks *(continued)*

The Well Versed (15+ years)			
85.	Christopher M. Graham	04/16/89	Wilton, CT, attorney, 44
86.	Jay A. Schrader	11/28/89	Springdale, PA, retiree, 61
87.	Hal Gensler	12/04/89	New River, AZ, retiree, 62
88T.	John H. Wallace, Jr.	12/31/89	Ishpeming, MI, photographer, 58
88T.	John H. Wallace, III	12/31/89	Seattle, WA, website developer, 32
88T.	Mark Washburne	12/31/89	Mendham, NJ, professor, 52
91.	Tomas Loughead	07/07/90	Huntsville, AL, engineer, 68
92.	John C. Roemer, III	08/01/90	Parkton, MD, education, 70 *
93.	Richard J. Wright	08/03/90	Pittsburgh, PA, track & cross-country coach, 57
94.	John Wolff	09/01/90	Spotsylvania, VA, banker, 57
95.	Ted Sabinas	12/08/90	Cedar Springs, MI, teacher/coach, 56
96.	John L. Faz	12/26/90	Lincoln, NE, police officer, 55
97T.	Patrick L. Steele	12/30/90	Adel, IA, vice president, 55
97T.	Jeff L. Morgan	12/30/90	Reston, VA, IT trainer, 52
99.	Ronald J. Landrum	01/01/91	San Jose, CA, zoologist, 58
100.	Matthew J. Ketterman	07/01/91	Greensboro, NC, business owner, 37
101.	Danny Sullivan	07/12/91	San Carlos, CA, restaurateur, 59
102.	William E. Chatman	07/23/91	Brooksville, FL, teacher/coach, 59
103.	Patrick J. Foley	08/30/91	Northfield, MN, retiree, 60 *
104.	David N. Potter	01/01/92	Ashland, OH, retiree, 56
105.	Mark T. Wigler	07/07/92	Hubbardston, MA, director, 60
106.	Gabrielle Cohen	11/10/92	Petrolia, CA, theatre production, 46
107.	Edwin N. Dupree	06/23/93	Faith, NC, retiree, 67
108.	Stanley Weissman	09/30/93	Miami Beach, FL, retiree, 68
The Experienced (10+ years)			
109.	Jeffrey Sider	01/01/94	Plainview, NY, orthopedic surgeon, 52
110.	Joel Pearson	09/03/94	Ferndale, WA, college track coach, 23
111.	Scott Fodstad	04/12/95	Crystal, MN, mail handler, 53
112.	John Nikolic	04/29/95	Pearl, MS, real estate manager, 66
113.	Larry Albertson	06/09/95	Ballwin, MO, production technician, 57
114.	Richard J. Kerr	07/30/95	Kokomo, IN, pipe fitter/bus driver, 53 *
115.	A. F. DeYoung, Jr.	11/08/96	Woodland Hills, CA, photographer, 62
116.	Stephen J. Gurdak	11/21/96	Springfield, VA, police detective, 53
117.	Karen Queally	01/01/97	Millbrae, CA, physical therapist, 56 *
118.	Grant Woodman	10/06/97	Ithaca, MI, college administrator, 34 *
119.	Thomas B. Welch	01/01/98	Eden Prairie, MN, portfolio manager, 52
120.	Howard P. Feldman	01/13/98	St. Louis, MO, retiree, 57 *

121.	Thomas W. Whitely	01/16/98	Fair Lawn, NJ, PE teacher, 50
122T.	Debbie Ciccati	04/01/98	San Diego, CA, educator, 53
122T.	Craig B. Snapp	04/01/98	El Cajon, CA, retiree, 58 *
124.	Weldon K. Burton	07/14/98	Fort Walton Beach, FL, retiree, 49
The Proficient (5+ years)			
125.	Andrew S. McPherson	08/16/99	Palatine, IL, business owner, 44
126.	Jeffrey Shumway	10/09/99	Provo, UT, professor, 55
127.	Diane Shumway	05/27/00	Provo, UT, retiree, 53
128.	Margaret Sherrod	06/02/00	Millersville, MD, teacher, 53
129.	Susan L. Jones	01/01/01	Boys Ranch, TX, administrative assistant, 44
130.	Patrick W. Sinopoli	01/26/01	Turtle Creek, PA, construction manager, 56
131.	Ronald W. Shealy	04/01/01	Lexington, SC, field supervisor, 62 *
132.	Kevin Rison	09/14/01	Orlando, FL, human resource manager, 37
133.	Jane E. Hefferan	10/27/01	Nashville, TN, law student, 27
134.	James R. Merritt	10/29/01	Buford, GA, delivery driver, 61
135.	Ralph Edwards	04/07/02	Des Moines, IA, assistant principal, 61 *
136.	Mercedes M. Murolo	05/04/02	Santa Rosa, CA, artist/ad executive, 58 *
137.	Terrell Worley	05/05/02	Rancho Cucamonga, CA, case worker, 48 *
138.	George A. Hancock	06/22/02	Windber, PA, education, 55 *
139.	Eliza Eshelman	09/21/02	Columbia City, IN, student, 23
140.	Roger D. Raymond	11/15/02	Marco Island, FL, music store owner, 57
141.	Ken Johnson	12/28/02	Huntsville, TX, retiree, 67 *
142.	Vincent Attanucci	01/08/03	The Woodlands, TX, engineer, 55
143.	Andrew Feravich	10/21/03	Cedar Springs, MI, student, 19
The Neophytes (1+ years)			
144.	Joseph K. Booth	05/03/04	Bothell, WA, land planner, 31
145.	Ed Reid	05/27/04	Bradenton, FL, builder, 49
146.	Neil Scott	06/02/04	Seattle, WA, sports reporter, 62 *
147.	Prince Whatley	07/01/04	Birmingham, AL, sales, 40
148.	Veronica V. Rust	07/22/04	Palm Springs, CA, office manager, 28
149T.	Vivian Wilson	10/11/04	Short Hills, NJ, physician, 49
149T.	Howard Kaplan	10/11/04	Madison, WI, philosopher, 30
151.	Nancy L. Harmon	01/01/05	Berwick, PA, fitness director, 49
152.	Susan Ruzicka	07/09/05	Harrison City, PA, A/R specialist, 45
153.	Timothy J. Eshelman	07/24/05	Roanoke, IN, sales, 48
154.	Peter T. Eshelman, Jr.	07/27/05	Columbia City, IN, insurance, 55
155.	Jason Morgan	08/14/05	Bradenton, FL, human resources, 39
156.	D. Scott Cyphers	08/29/05	Bedford, MA, research scientist, 48
157.	Don Slusser	09/10/05	Monroeville, PA, teacher, 57 *

(continued)

Official List of Active U.S. Running Streaks *(continued)*

The Neophytes (1+ years) *(continued)*			
158.	Rick Stern	09/21/05	Round Rock, TX, financial advisor, 60
159.	Karen J. Wallace	09/26/05	Ishpeming, MI, clerical, 53 *
160.	Pete Gilman	11/06/05	Rochester, MN, correctional sergeant, 33
161.	Duncan Cameron	12/06/05	Palm Harbor, FL, compliance officer, 66 *
162.	Daniel J. Dugan, Jr.	12/30/05	Howell, NJ, police officer, 51
163.	Gary R. Scott	01/19/06	Olathe, KS, teacher, 58
164.	David S. Duncan, III	06/03/06	McKenzie, TN, assistant principal/coach, 51
165.	Darrin D. Young	06/24/06	Columbia, MO, sales, 42 *
166T.	Homer Hastings	07/01/06	Newcastle, WY, teacher, 65 *
166T.	Michael McDonell	07/01/06	Seattle, WA, psychologist, 32
168.	Michael Dallas	08/07/06	Norwich, UK, Air Force civilian, 45
169.	Brad Kautz	08/20/06	Rochester, MN, occupational therapist, 51
170.	Scott J. Palm	09/09/06	Chaumont, NY, Army civilian, 44
171.	Don Brakebill	09/29/06	Bakersfield, CA, jeweler, 61
172.	Thomas A. Fons	11/10/06	Katy, TX, stockbroker, 42
173.	David McMain	11/11/06	Brandon, MS, claims adjustor, 51
174T.	William D. Nelson	12/15/06	Houston, TX, business, 43 *
174T.	Heather E. Nelson	12/15/06	Houston, TX, student, 17
176.	Doug Hubred	12/23/06	Golden Valley, MN, teacher, 40
177.	Beth Casavant	12/26/06	Northbridge, MA, homemaker, 35
178T.	Freddy Reyes	01/01/07	Sinking Springs, PA, JROTC instructor, 45
178T.	William T. Donahoo	01/01/07	Aurora, CO, physician, 45
178T.	Stephanie Mera	01/01/07	Redlands, CA, student, 20
181.	Rene G. Burgess	01/03/07	Boiling Springs, PA, U.S. Army, 46
182.	Bill Street	02/10/07	Tucson, AZ, computer consultant, 40
183.	Nevertha R. Brooks	03/08/07	Chicago, IL, accounting associate, 37
184.	Yvette Faris	03/15/07	Wallingford, CT, IT director, 48
185.	David M. Woodson	06/25/07	Newport News, VA, student, 21
186.	Corey A. Escue	07/15/07	Chicago, IL, missionary, 35
187.	Geza Feld	08/01/07	Farmingdale, NY, retiree, 75 *
188.	Kevin Brunson	10/06/07	Reno, NV, insurance agent, 49
189.	Ellen S. Runnoe	11/03/07	Wausau, WI, teacher, 54 *

* Indicates listing on both the active and retired running streak lists.

Reprinted, by permission, from U.S. Running Streak Association, Inc., 2008, "Official U.S.A. active running streak list." [Online]. Available: http://runeveryday.com/lists/RunningStreakList.htm (February 11, 2009).

Official List of Retired U.S. Running Streaks (as certified by the United States Running Streak Association, December 1, 2008)

		Start date – End date	Length of streak	Hometown
1.	Robert C. Ray	04/04/67 – 04/07/05	13,844 days (38 years, 5 days)	Baltimore, MD
2.	Ronald Kmiec	11/28/75 – 11/26/07	11,687 days (31 years, 364 days)	Carlisle, MA
3.	Geza Feld	10/01/76 – 07/27/07	11,257 days (30 years, 300 days)	Farmingdale, NY *
4.	Lawrence E. Sundberg	01/01/77 – 12/31/06	10,957 days (30 years, 0 days)	Farmington, CT
5.	James R. Scarborough	07/09/79 – 07/09/08	10,594 days (29 years, 1 day)	Rancho Palos Verdes, CA
6.	Larry Baldasari, Sr.	01/08/78 – 04/03/06	10,313 days (28 years, 86 days)	Hamilton Square, NJ
7.	Fred Winkel	12/20/79 – 07/27/07	10,082 days (27 years, 220 days)	Glen Hood, NY
8.	J. Patrick Growney	01/01/80 – 06/21/07	10,036 days (27 years, 174 days)	Lavallette, NJ
9.	Joseph B. Hyder	04/04/79 – 09/11/06	10,023 days (27 years, 161 days)	Black Mountain, NC
10.	Don Slusser	01/03/72 – 06/11/99	10,022 days (27 years, 160 days)	Monroeville, PA *
11.	Diana L. Nelson	01/11/82 – 10/02/07	9,396 days (25 years, 265 days)	Dixon, IL
12.	Mike McAvoy	05/17/81 – 01/21/07	9,381 days (25 years, 250 days)	Duluth, MN
13.	Roger H. Nelson	08/01/81 – 02/27/07	9,342 days (25 years, 211 days)	Colleyville, TX
14.	Robert L. Bartz	05/01/79 – 08/22/04	9,246 days (25 years, 115 days)	Phoenix, AZ
15.	Kevin Simons	09/20/82 – 06/24/07	9,044 days (24 years, 278 days)	Hampton, MA
16.	George A. Hancock	02/26/78 – 05/24/02	8,854 days (24 years, 88 days)	Windber, PA *
17.	Robert Aby	02/12/83 – 01/03/07	8,727 days (23 years, 326 days)	Worthington, MN
18.	Norman Grimmett	05/07/78 – 03/21/02	8,720 days (23 years, 319 days)	San Antonio, TX
19.	Kenneth J. Roth	07/28/81 – 05/28/05	8,706 days (23 years, 305 days)	Del Mar, CA
20.	Sue S. Favor	12/20/84 – 05/03/08	8,524 days (23 years, 136 days)	Downey, CA
21.	Jay Kammerzell	01/01/83 – 01/10/06	8,411 days (23 years, 10 days)	Everett, WA
22.	Allan S. Field	09/20/80 – 03/28/03	8,225 days (22 years, 190 days)	Columbia, MD
23.	Richard B. Patterson	02/20/87 – 09/24/08	7,888 days (21 years, 218 days)	El Paso, TX
24.	Homer Hastings	09/08/84 – 12/31/05	7,785 days (21 years, 115 days)	Newcastle, WY *
25.	Len S. Burton	06/28/83 – 09/17/04	7,753 days (21 years, 83 days)	Hot Springs Village, AR
26.	Peter Lefferts	01/26/81 – 02/18/02	7,694 days (21 years, 24 days)	Naples, FL
27.	Bob Hensley	12/02/74 – 06/02/94	7,123 days (19 years, 183 days)	Port St. Luci, FL
28.	Syl Pascale	12/22/78 – 06/17/97	6,753 days (18 years, 179 days)	San Carlos, CA
29.	Neil Scott	08/05/86 – 05/21/04	6,499 days (17 years, 291 days)	Seattle, WA *
30.	David L. Biersmith	09/08/84 – 05/22/02	6,466 days (17 years, 257 days)	Kansas City, MO
31.	Bob Reininger	03/01/81 – 07/07/98	6,338 days (17 years, 129 days)	Shelocta, PA

(continued)

32.	Ronnie O. Shaw	01/01/86 – 12/09/02	6,187 days (16 years, 343 days)	Fort Worth, TX
33.	Kenneth Vercammen	09/10/82 – 01/06/99	5,963 days (16 years, 119 days)	New Brunswick, NJ
34.	Ray Lorden	10/31/89 – 05/31/05	5,692 days (15 years, 213 days)	Parkville, MD
35.	John P. Flahie	03/14/84 – 06/14/99	5,571 days (15 years, 92 days)	Sylvania, OH
36.	Ralph Edwards	06/20/88 – 09/18/01	4,839 days (13 years, 91 days)	Des Moines, IA *
37.	John C. Roemer, III	12/27/77 – 06/28/90	4,567 days (12 years, 184 days)	Parkton, MD *
38.	Bob Hensley	07/02/94 – 12/06/06	4,541 days (12 years, 158 days)	Port St. Luci, FL
39.	Stephen C. Moosbrugger	12/31/94 – 12/31/06	4,384 days (12 years, 1 day)	Edina, MN
40.	David T. Lloyd	12/11/91 – 12/31/02	4,039 days (11 years, 21 days)	Fort Worth, TX
41.	Stephen Gould	04/30/94 – 05/12/04	3,666 days (10 years, 14 days)	Lincolnville, ME
42.	Thomas Damoulakis	01/01/90 – 12/31/99	3,652 days (10 years, 0 days)	Wilbraham, MA
43.	Daniel R. Sheeran	12/23/86 – 11/20/96	3,621 days (9 years, 334 days)	Orange, CA
44.	Fred H. Kameny	07/23/95 – 12/16/04	3,435 days (9 years, 148 days)	Chapel Hill, NC
45.	Terrell Worley	04/03/93 – 11/21/01	3,154 days (8 years, 230 days)	Rancho Cucamonga, CA *
46.	Mercedes M. Murolo	12/25/91 – 04/28/02	3,047 days (8 years, 125 days)	Santa Rosa, CA *
47.	Herbert L. Fred	08/01/70 – 05/27/78	2,857 days (7 years, 300 days)	Houston, TX
48.	Robert M. Crosby, Jr.	12/22/99 – 07/29/07	2,777 days (7 years, 220 days)	Summerville, SC
49.	Kenneth Vercammen	03/14/99 – 05/21/06	2,626 days (7 years, 69 days)	New Brunswick, NJ
50.	Ronald Whittemore	01/02/89 – 02/28/96	2,614 days (7 years, 57 days)	Claremont, NH
51.	Richard Holmes	07/29/98 – 05/23/05	2,491 days (6 years, 300 days)	Durham, NC
52.	Wendell J. DeBoer	06/22/80 – 12/31/86	2,384 days (6 years, 193 days)	Falcon Heights, MN
53.	Ben Zappa	12/09/87 – 05/07/04	2,342 days (6 years, 150 days)	Ridgeway, PA
54.	David L. DeBoer	07/10/72 – 08/12/78	2,225 days (6 years, 34 days)	Manchester, MO
55.	Paul E. Boyette	06/02/02 – 06/16/08	2,207 days (6 years, 15 days)	Chesapeake, VA
56.	Ralph Edwards	02/14/82 – 02/22/88	2,200 days (6 years, 9 days)	Des Moines, IA *
57.	Mary Roemer	08/01/81 – 06/14/87	2,144 days (5 years, 318 days)	Parkton, MD
58.	Ronald K. Kallinen	01/24/99 – 08/17/04	2,033 days (5 years, 207 days)	Katy, TX
59.	William J. Benton	03/09/70 – 09/03/75	2,005 days (5 years, 179 days)	Farmington Hills, MI *
60.	Richard J. Kerr	12/25/86 – 06/15/92	2,000 days (5 years, 174 days)	Kokomo, IN *
61.	James C. Bates	11/18/00 – 04/07/06	1,967 days (5 years, 141 days)	Hampton, VA
62.	Bob Hensley	11/06/69 – 11/30/74	1,851 days (5 years, 25 days)	Port St. Luci, FL
63.	Grant Woodman	09/02/92 – 08/29/97	1,823 days (4 years, 362 days)	Ithaca, MI *
64.	Ken Johnson	12/30/97 – 12/14/02	1,811 days (4 years, 350 days)	Huntsville, TX *
65.	Jay Kammerzell	07/16/74 – 03/31/79	1,720 days (4 years, 259 days)	Everett, WA

66.	Mark K. Hall	12/27/92 – 08/18/97	1,696 days (4 years, 235 days)	Dallas, TX
67.	Stephen R. Minagil	12/27/94 – 01/24/99	1,551 days (4 years, 90 days)	Las Vegas, NV
68.	Mark K. Hall	05/17/01 – 08/10/05	1,547 days (4 years, 86 days)	Dallas, TX
69.	Fred H. Kameny	10/03/81 – 12/19/85	1,539 days (4 years, 78 days)	Chapel Hill, NC
70.	Karen Queally	01/01/91 – 12/31/94	1,461 days (4 years, 1 day)	Millbrae, CA *
71.	Don Slusser	02/14/00 – 11/04/03	1,360 days (3 years, 264 days)	Monroeville, PA *
72.	Patrick J. Foley	06/11/87 – 02/13/91	1,344 days (3 years, 248 days)	Northfield, MN *
73.	Ronald W. Shealy	07/15/89 – 02/25/93	1,322 days (3 years, 226 days)	Lexington, SC *
74.	Pete Lefferts	03/08/02 – 08/02/05	1,244 days (3 years, 148 days)	Glenside, PA
75.	Herbert L. Fred	02/12/04 – 02/06/07	1,091 days (2 years, 360 days)	Houston, TX
76.	Paige Pearson	08/28/02 – 06/17/05	1,025 days (2 years, 295 days)	Mead, WA
77.	Jay Kammerzell	01/23/06 – 11/06/08	1,019 days (2 years, 289 days)	Everett, WA
78.	Terrell Worley	08/03/90 – 03/27/93	985 days (2 years, 255 days)	Rancho Cucamonga, CA *
79.	Richard Holmes	07/23/05 – 02/19/08	942 days (2 years, 212 days)	Durham, NC
80.	Richard Holmes	11/14/95 – 05/27/98	926 days (2 years, 196 days)	Durham, NC
81.	Wendell J. DeBoer	02/18/78 – 06/20/80	854 days (2 years, 124 days)	Falcon Heights, MN
82.	Norman Grimmett	12/16/04 – 03/20/07	825 days (2 years, 95 days)	San Antonio, TX
83.	William D. Nelson	09/01/79 – 10/20/81	781 days (2 years, 50 days)	Houston, TX *
84.	Ronnie O. Shaw	01/01/82 – 01/18/84	748 days (2 years, 18 days)	Fort Worth, TX
85.	Stephen Gould	08/30/04 – 09/13/06	745 days (2 years, 15 days)	Lincolnville, ME
86.	Wendell J. DeBoer	01/02/87 – 12/27/88	726 days (1 year, 361 days)	Falcon Heights, MN
87.	Duncan Cameron	12/03/02 – 10/09/04	677 days (1 year, 312 days)	Palm Harbor, FL *
88.	Howard P. Feldman	04/01/96 – 01/07/98	647 days (1 year, 282 days)	St. Louis, MO *
89.	Ken Johnson	01/01/92 – 08/22/93	600 days (1 year, 235 days)	Huntsville, TX *
90.	Karen J. Wallace	01/01/04 – 08/09/05	587 days (1 year, 222 days)	Ishpeming, MI *
91.	Eileen Dibler	02/02/02 – 09/07/03	583 days (1 year, 218 days)	Columbia, MD
92.	Ronald Kmiec	04/19/74 – 11/16/75	577 days (1 year, 212 days)	Carlisle, MA
93.	Terrell Worley	09/05/82 – 02/28/84	541 days (1 year, 176 days)	Rancho Cucamonga, CA *
94.	Liz Schecter	12/03/06 – 04/18/08	503 days (1 year, 138 days)	Kinnelon, NJ
95.	Ellen S. Runnoe	04/06/06 – 08/06/07	488 days (1 year, 123 days)	Wausau, WI *
96.	Craig B. Snapp	12/22/78 – 04/21/80	487 days (1 year, 122 days)	El Cajon, CA *
97.	Ronald W. Shealy	04/23/88 – 07/13/89	447 days (1 year, 82 days)	Lexington, SC *
98.	Perry Romanowski	01/15/07 – 04/03/08	445 days (1 year, 80 days)	Chicago, IL
99.	Ronnie O. Shaw	05/15/07 – 07/31/08	444 days (1 year, 78 days)	Fort Worth, TX
100.	Stephen G. Bardsley	01/01/07 – 02/19/08	415 days (1 year, 50 days)	Stevensville, MD
101.	Cindy Lefferts	03/05/03 – 04/15/04	408 days (1 year, 43 days)	Naples, FL

(continued)

Official List of Retired U.S. Running Streaks *(continued)*

102.	Patrick J. Foley	12/23/79 – 01/08/81	383 days (1 year, 18 days)	Northfield, MN *
103.	Peter Eshelman, Jr.	12/15/06 – 01/01/08	383 days (1 year, 18 days)	Columbia City, IN
104.	Darrin D. Young	01/01/97 – 01/16/98	381 days (1 year, 16 days)	Columbia, MD *
105.	Barry Abrahams	12/20/76 – 12/28/77	374 days (1 year, 9 days)	Lincoln, NE *
106.	Tammy M. Root	01/01/07 – 01/02/08	367 days (1 year, 2 days)	Richmond, IN
107.	Chris J. DeLeon	07/03/07 – 07/03/08	367 days (1 year, 1 day)	Wichita, KS
108.	John Granger	01/01/05 – 01/01/06	366 days (1 year, 1 day)	Port Hadlock, WA
109.	Teri Davison	08/04/06 – 08/04/07	366 days (1 year, 1 day)	Leander, TX
110.	Karen Queallev	01/01/86 – 12/31/86	365 days (1 year, 0 days)	Millbrae, CA *
111.	Heather L. Bagan	12/31/06 – 12/30/07	365 days (1 year, 0 days)	Los Angeles, CA
112.	Tiffany A. Brigner	01/01/07 – 12/31/07	365 days (1 year, 0 days)	Lakeland, CO

* Indicates listing on both the active and retired running streak lists.

Reprinted, by permission, from U.S. Running Streak Association, Inc., 2008, "Official U.S.A. retired running streak list." [Online]. Available: http://runeveryday.com/lists/RetiredStreakList.htm (February 11, 2009).

References and Bibliography

PROLOGUE

Centers for Disease Control and Prevention. 2006. Percentage of adults 18 years and over who engaged in regular leisure-time physical activity: United States, 1997-2005. www.cdc.gov/nchs/data/nhis/earlyrelease/200606_07.pdf.

———. 2008. The U.S. is on the brink of a longevity revolution. www.cdc.gov/aging.

Chakravarty, E.F., H.B. Hubert, V.B. Lingala, and J.F. Fries. 2008. Reduce disability and mortality among aging runners. *Archives of Internal Medicine* 168(15): 1638-1646.

Melov, S., M.A. Tarnopolsky, K. Beckman, K. Felkey, and A. Hubbard. 2007. Resistance exercise reverses aging in human skeletal muscle. *Science Daily*. www.sciencedaily.com/releases/2007/05/070522210936.htm.

U.S. Census Bureau. August 9, 2006. Facts for features. www.census.gov/Press-Release/www/releases/archives/facts_for_features_special_editions/007276.html.

CHAPTER 1

DiNubile, N. 2005. *Framework: Your 7-step program for healthy muscles, bones, and joints*. New York: Rodale.

Le, P. September 9, 2000. Faith Ireland says she had baby at 22. *Seattle Post-Intelligencer.*

Postman, D. October 29, 1998. Ireland, Foley sport polar-opposite styles. *Seattle Times.*

Tolle, E. 2004. *The power of now: A guide to spiritual enlightenment*. Novato, CA: New World Library.

Westcott, W.L., and T.R. Baechle. 2007. *Strength training past 50*. Champaign, IL: Human Kinetics.

CHAPTER 2

Brandt, R., and T. Weisel. 2003. *Capital instincts: Life as an entrepreneur, financier, and athlete.* Hoboken, NJ: Wiley.

CHAPTER 3

McConica, J. November 1, 2004. Jim McConica recounts his toughest swim: From Catalina to the U.S. mainland. *Swimming World.*

Stager, J.M., J.D. Johnston, L.D. Raisbeck, & F.J. Benay. 2005. Biological markers of aging in highly active adults. *Medicine & Science in Sports & Exercise* 37(5): S255.

Whitten, P. March 2005. Holding back the years: How much should we decline with age? *Swimming World.*

Wu, A. January 1, 2007. Reconnecting with his passion: Greg Shaw, ex-hippie, talks about his latest race. *Swimming World.*

CHAPTER 4

Centers for Disease Control and Prevention. April 25, 2008. Falls among older adults: An overview. http://cdc.gov/ncipc/factsheets/adultfalls.htm.

Vad, V., and H. Hinzmann. 2004. *Back Rx: A 15-minute-a-day yoga- and Pilates-based program to end low back pain.* New York: Gotham Books.

CHAPTER 5

Agency for Healthcare Research and Quality. 2007. Healthcare cost and utilization project facts and figures: Statistics on hospital-based care in the United States in 2005. Rockville, MD: Author. www.hcup-us.ahrq.gov/reports.jsp.

American College of Sports Medicine. 1998. Position stand on exercise and physical activity for older adults. *Medicine & Science in Sports & Exercise* 30(6): 992-1008.

Bass, C. 1980. *Ripped: The sensible way to achieve ultimate muscularity.* Albuquerque: Ripped Enterprises.

———. 1984. *The lean advantage.* Albuquerque: Ripped Enterprises.

———. 2007. *Great expectations: Health, fitness, leanness without suffering.* Albuquerque: Ripped Enterprises.

Cooper, K. 1968. *Aerobics.* New York: Evans.

Spirduso, W.W. 1995. *Physical dimensions of aging.* Champaign, IL: Human Kinetics.

Weil, A. 2005. *Healthy aging: A lifelong guide to your well-being.* New York: Anchor Books.

CHAPTER 6

Haney, B. (Producer). 2004. *Racing against the clock.* [Documentary film.] Uncommon Productions.

CHAPTER 7

Associated Press. March 24, 2002. He lives to run and he runs for his life. *New York Times.*

Karnazes, D. 2005. *Ultramarathon man: Confessions of an all-night runner.* New York: Tarcher.

Kuehls, D. March 2003. Triumph of the heart. *Runner's World.*

MacGregor, S. May 7, 1999. A survivor's now thriving. *Cincinnati Enquirer.*

Starr, C. May 3, 2001. Runner's renewal. *Cincinnati Post.*

CHAPTER 8

Amdur, N. April 20, 1982. Salazar Wins Fastest Boston Marathon. *New York Times.*

Stein, J. October 15, 2007. Finishing strong. *Los Angeles Times.*

CHAPTER 9

Bergquist, L. August 8, 2006. It's a long run: Bay man hasn't missed a daily run in 25 years—and is as passionate as ever. *Milwaukee Journal Sentinel.*

Chakravarty, E.F., H.B. Hubert, V.B. Lingala, E. Zatarain, and J.F. Fries. August 2008. Long distance running and knee osteoarthritis: A prospective study. *American Journal of Preventive Medicine* 35(2).

CHAPTER 10

Hearts and records broken. April 28, 1952. *Life.*

Mueller, L. (Producer). 1987. *Silver into gold.* [Documentary film.]

Morales, T. July/August 2003. Portrait of a grand master. *Swim Magazine.*

Schollander, D., and D. Savage. 1971. *Deep water.* New York: Crown.

CHAPTER 11

Auerbach. S. (Producer). 2005. *Race Across America.* [Television broadcast on NBC.]

Nichols, J.F., J.E. Palmer, and S.S. Levy. 2003. Low bone mineral density in highly trained male master cyclists. *Osteoporosis International* 14(8): 644-649.

CHAPTER 12

Brendle, D.C., L.J.O. Joseph, J.D. Sorkin, D. McNelly, and L.I. Katzel. 2003. Aging and marathon times in an 81-year-old man who competed in 591 marathons. *American Journal of Cardiology* 91(9): 1154-1156.

Cooper, K. 1968. *Aerobics.* New York: Evans.

Index